Dietary Reference Intakes Proposed Definition of Dietary Fiber

A Report of the
Panel on the Definition of Dietary Fiber
and the
Standing Committee on the Scientific Evaluation of Dietary
Reference Intakes
Food and Nutrition Board
INSTITUTE OF MEDICINE

NATIONAL ACADEMY PRESS
Washington, D.C.

NATIONAL ACADEMY PRESS 2101 Constitution Avenue, N.W. Washington, DC 20418

NOTICE: The project that is the subject of this report was approved by the Governing Board of the National Research Council, whose members are drawn from the councils of the National Academy of Sciences, the National Academy of Engineering, and the Institute of Medicine. The members of the committee responsible for the report were chosen for their special competences and with regard for appropriate balance.

Support for this project was provided by Health Canada; U.S. Department of Health and Human Services Office of Disease Prevention and Health Promotion, Contract No. 282-96-0033, TO4; the Dietary Reference Intakes Private Foundation Fund, including the Dannon Institute and the International Life Sciences Institute; and the Dietary Reference Intakes Corporate Donors' Fund. Contributors to the Fund to date include Daiichi Fine Chemicals, Inc.; Kemin Foods, L.C.; M&M/Mars; Mead Johnson Nutritionals; Nabisco Foods Group; Natural Source Vitamin E Association; Roche Vitamins Inc.; U.S. Borax; and Weider Nutrition Group. The opinions or conclusions expressed herein are those of the committee and do not necessarily reflect those of the funders.

International Standard Book No. 0-309-07564-5
This report is available for sale from the National Academy Press, 2101 Constitution Avenue, N.W., Box 285, Washington, DC 20055; call (800) 624-6242 or (202) 334-3313 (in the Washington metropolitan area), or visit the NAP's online bookstore at **http://www.nap.edu**.

For more information about the Institute of Medicine or the Food and Nutrition Board, visit the IOM home page at **http://www.iom.edu**.
Copyright 2001 by the National Academy of Sciences. All rights reserved.

Printed in the United States of America

"Knowing is not enough; we must apply, Willing is not enough; we must do."

—Goethe

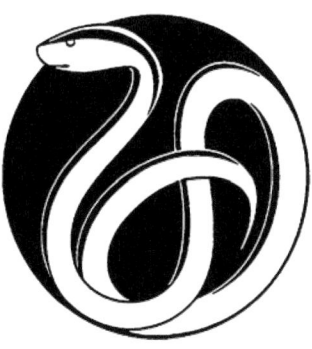

INSTITUTE OF MEDICINE
Shaping the Future for Health

THE NATIONAL ACADEMIES

National Academy of Sciences
National Academy of Engineering
Institute of Medicine
National Research Council

The **National Academy of Sciences** is a private, nonprofit, self-perpetuating society of distinguished scholars engaged in scientific and engineering research, dedicated to the furtherance of science and technology and to their use for the general welfare. Upon the authority of the charter granted to it by the Congress in 1863, the Academy has a mandate that requires it to advise the federal government on scientific and technical matters. Dr. Bruce M. Alberts is president of the National Academy of Sciences.

The **National Academy of Engineering** was established in 1964, under the charter of the National Academy of Sciences, as a parallel organization of outstanding engineers. It is autonomous in its administration and in the selection of its members, sharing with the National Academy of Sciences the responsibility for advising the federal government. The National Academy of Engineering also sponsors engineering programs aimed at meeting national needs, encourages education and research, and recognizes the superior achievements of engineers. Dr. William. A. Wulf is president of the National Academy of Engineering.

The **Institute of Medicine** was established in 1970 by the National Academy of Sciences to secure the services of eminent members of appropriate professions in the examination of policy matters pertaining to the health of the public. The Institute acts under the responsibility given to the National Academy of Sciences by its congressional charter to be an adviser to the federal government and, upon its own initiative, to identify issues of medical care, research, and education. Dr. Kenneth I. Shine is president of the Institute of Medicine.

The **National Research Council** was organized by the National Academy of Sciences in 1916 to associate the broad community of science and technology with the Academy's purposes of furthering knowledge and advising the federal government. Functioning in accordance with general policies determined by the Academy, the Council has become the principal operating agency of both the National Academy of Sciences and the National Academy of Engineering in providing services to the government, the public, and the scientific and engineering communities. The Council is administered jointly by both Academies and the Institute of Medicine. Dr. Bruce M. Alberts and Dr. William. A. Wulf are chairman and vice chairman, respectively, of the National Research Council.

www.national-academies.org

PANEL ON THE DEFINITION OF DIETARY FIBER

JOANNE R. LUPTON (chair), Faculty of Nutrition, Texas A&M University, College Station
GEORGE C. FAHEY, Department of Animal Sciences, University of Illinois at Urbana-Champaign
DAVID A. JENKINS, Department of Nutritional Sciences, University of Toronto, Ontario
JUDITH A. MARLETT, Department of Nutritional Science, University of Wisconsin-Madison
JOANNE L. SLAVIN, Department of Food Science and Nutrition, University of Minnesota, St. Paul
JON A. STORY, Department of Foods and Nutrition, Purdue University, West Lafayette, Indiana
CHRISTINE L. WILLIAMS, Department of Pediatrics, Columbia University, Babies and Children's Hospital of New York

Consultants

LEON PROSKY, Prosky Associates, Rockville, Maryland
ALISON M. STEPHEN, CANTOX Health Sciences International, Mississauga, Ontario

Staff

PAULA R. TRUMBO, Study Director
CARRIE L. HOLLOWAY, Research Assistant
MICHELE RAMSEY, Senior Project Assistant

STANDING COMMITTEE ON THE SCIENTIFIC EVALUATION OF DIETARY REFERENCE INTAKES

VERNON R. YOUNG (chair), Laboratory of Human Nutrition, School of Science, Massachusetts Institute of Technology, Cambridge

JOHN W. ERDMAN, JR. (vice chair), Division of Nutritional Sciences, College of Agriculture, Consumer and Environmental Sciences, University of Illinois at Urbana-Champaign

LINDSAY H. ALLEN, Department of Nutrition, University of California at Davis

STEPHANIE A. ATKINSON, Department of Pediatrics, Faculty of Health Sciences, McMaster University, Hamilton, Ontario

ROBERT J. COUSINS, Center for Nutritional Sciences, University of Florida, Gainesville

JOHANNA T. DWYER, Frances Stern Nutrition Center, New England Medical Center and Tufts University, Boston, Massachusetts

JOHN D. FERNSTROM, UPMC Health System Weight Management Center, University of Pittsburgh School of Medicine, Pennsylvania

SCOTT M. GRUNDY, Center for Human Nutrition, University of Texas Southwestern Medical Center at Dallas

SANFORD A. MILLER, Center for Food and Nutrition Policy, Georgetown University, Washington, D.C.

WILLIAM M. RAND, Department of Family Medicine and Community Health, Tufts University School of Medicine, Boston, Massachusetts

U.S. Government Liaison

KATHRYN McMURRY, Office of Disease Prevention and Health Promotion, U.S. Department of Health and Human Services, Washington, D.C.

Canadian Government Liaison

PETER W.F. FISCHER, Nutrition Research Division, Health Protection Branch, Health Canada, Ottawa

Staff

ALLISON A. YATES, Study Director
GAIL E. SPEARS, Administrative Assistant
MARY POOS, Senior Program Officer
SANDRA SCHLICKER, Senior Program Officer
PAULA R. TRUMBO, Senior Program Officer
KIMBERLY FREITAG, Research Associate
ALICE L. VOROSMARTI, Research Associate
CARRIE L. HOLLOWAY, Research Assistant
SHELLEY GOLDBERG, Senior Project Assistant

FOOD AND NUTRITION BOARD

CUTBERTO GARZA (chair), Division of Nutrition, Cornell University, Ithaca, New York

ALFRED H. MERRILL, JR. (vice chair), Department of Biochemistry and Center for Nutrition and Health Sciences, Emory University, Atlanta, Georgia

ROBERT M. RUSSELL (vice chair), Jean Mayer USDA Human Nutrition Research Center on Aging, Tufts University, Boston, Massachusetts

VIRGINIA A. STALLINGS (vice chair), Division of Gastroenterology and Nutrition, The Children's Hospital of Philadelphia, Pennsylvania

LARRY R. BEUCHAT, Center for Food Safety and Quality Enhancement, University of Georgia, Griffin

BENJAMIN CABALLERO, Center for Human Nutrition, Johns Hopkins University School of Hygiene and Public Health, Baltimore, Maryland

ROBERT J. COUSINS, Center for Nutritional Sciences, University of Florida, Gainesville

SHIRIKI KUMANYIKA, Center for Clinical Epidemiology and Biostatistics, University of Pennsylvania School of Medicine, Philadelphia

LYNN PARKER, Child Nutrition Programs and Nutrition Policy, Food Research and Action Center, Washington, D.C.

ROSS L. PRENTICE, Division of Public Health Sciences, Fred Hutchinson Cancer Research Center, Seattle, Washington

A. CATHARINE ROSS, Department of Nutrition, The Pennsylvania State University, University Park

ROBERT E. SMITH, R.E. Smith Consulting, Inc., Newport, Vermont

STEVE L. TAYLOR, Department of Food Science and Technology and Food Processing Center, University of Nebraska, Lincoln

IOM Liaison

JOHANNA T. DWYER, Frances Stern Nutrition Center, New England Medical Center and Tufts University, Boston, Massachusetts

Staff

ALLISON A. YATES, Director
GAIL E. SPEARS, Administrative Assistant
ALISON GROGAN, Financial Associate

REVIEWERS

This report has been reviewed in draft form by individuals chosen for their diverse perspectives and technical expertise, in accordance with procedures approved by the NRC's Report Review Committee. The purpose of this independent review is to provide candid and critical comments that will assist the institution in making its published report as sound as possible and to ensure that the report meets institutional standards for objectivity, evidence, and responsiveness to the study charge. The review comments and draft manuscript remain confidential to protect the integrity of the deliberative process. We wish to thank the following individuals for their review of this report: Nils-Georg Asp, Lund University, Sweden; Fergus Clydesdale, University of Massachusetts at Amherst; Martin Eastwood, Western General Hospital, Edinburgh, Scotland; Betty Li, U.S. Department of Agriculture, Beltsville, Maryland; Michael McBurney, W.K. Kellogg Institute, Battle Creek, Michigan; and Irwin Rosenberg, Jean Mayer U.S. Department of Agriculture Human Nutrition Research Center on Aging, Tufts University, Boston, Massachusetts.

Although the reviewers listed above have provided many constructive comments and suggestions, they were not asked to endorse the conclusions or recommendations nor did they see the final draft of the report before its release. The review of this report was overseen by Judith Stern, University of California at Davis, who was responsible for making certain that an independent examination of this report was carried out in accordance with institutional procedures and that all review comments were carefully considered. Responsibility for the final content of this report rests entirely with the authoring committee and the institution.

Contents

I.	OVERVIEW AND CHARGE TO THE PANEL	1
II.	DEFINITIONS OF DIETARY FIBER	3
III.	ISSUES IN DEFINING DIETARY FIBER	12
IV.	PROPOSED DEFINITION OF DIETARY FIBER	22
V.	IMPACT OF THE DEFINITIONS OF DIETARY FIBER AND UNRESOLVED ISSUES	26
VI.	REFERENCES	34
APPENDIX A:	Acknowledgments	43
APPENDIX B:	Glossary	45
APPENDIX C:	Development and Evolution of Methods Used to Purify and Measure Dietary Fiber	49
APPENDIX D:	Determination of Energy Values for Fibers	63

Dietary Reference Intakes: Proposed Definition of Dietary Fiber

I.
OVERVIEW AND CHARGE TO THE PANEL

Currently, a variety of definitions of dietary fiber exist worldwide. Some definitions are based solely on one or more analytical methods for isolating dietary fiber, while others are physiologically based. For instance, in the United States dietary fiber is defined by a number of analytical methods that are accepted by the Association of Official Analytical Chemists International (AOAC) and these methods isolate nondigestible animal and plant carbohydrates. In Canada, however, a formal definition has been in place that recognizes nondigestible food of plant origin, but not of animal origin, as dietary fiber. As nutrition labeling becomes uniform throughout the world, it is recognized that a single definition of dietary fiber is needed. Furthermore, new products are being developed or isolated that behave like fiber, yet do not meet the traditional definitions of fiber, either analytically or physiologically. A lack of consensus among various international groups and organizations exists.

The current situation regarding labeling and defining dietary fiber in the United States and many other countries is arbitrary due to its reliance on analytical methods as opposed to an accurate definition that includes its role in health. Without an accurate definition, compounds can be designed or isolated and concentrated using the currently available methods, without necessarily providing beneficial health effects. Other compounds can be developed that are nondigestible and provide beneficial health effects, yet do not meet the current U.S. definition based on analytical methods. For the above reasons, the Food and Nutrition Board, under the oversight of the Standing Committee on the Scientific Evaluation of Dietary Reference Intakes, assembled a Panel on the Defini tion of Dietary Fiber to develop a proposed definition(s) of dietary fiber. This Panel held three meetings and a workshop.

The first task of the Panel was to review all current definitions of dietary fiber. These definitions are described in Section II, "Definitions of Dietary Fiber" and summarized in Table 1. In the process of reviewing the current definitions, the Panel noted major areas of difference among the definitions as to whether the following were included: animal carbohydrates, carbohydrates not recovered by alcohol precipitation, mono- and disaccharides, lignin, resistant starch, and whether the fiber had to be intact and naturally occurring in food. Some definitions are based on analytical methods for dietary fiber and these methods are reviewed in Table 2. Finally, some definitions require that a fiber have specific physiological effects, whereas others do not. How each current definition has dealt with these issues is summarized in Table 3. The Panel's analyses of each of these differentiating issues are found in section III, "Issues in Defining Dietary Fiber". Discussion and resolution of each of these differences among existing definitions formed the basis of the Panel's recommendation, which is described under section IV, "Proposed Definition of Dietary Fiber", together with an accompanying explanation for each aspect of the definition. Finally, section V, "Impact of the Definitions of Dietary Fiber and Unresolved Issues", delineates the likely consequences of adopting the proposed definitions with respect to their impact on: (1) analytical methodology, (2) recommended levels of intake, (3) food composi-tion databases, (4) dietary fiber research, (5) developments in the food industry, and (6) nutrition labeling.

Based on the Panel's deliberations, the following definitions are proposed:

Dietary Fiber consists of nondigestible carbohydrates and lignin that are intrinsic and intact in plants.

Added Fiber consists of isolated, nondigestible carbohydrates that have beneficial physiological effects in humans.

Total Fiber is the sum of *Dietary Fiber* and *Added Fiber.*

Following the release of these proposed definitions, it is expected that significant discussion will result in order to ascertain the extent to which they advance the move toward an acceptable framework for methodologically appropriate definitions based on the role of fiber in health. Comments regarding the acceptability of the proposed definitions and the framework for their incorporation into labeling and research initiatives are welcomed with the expectation that the definitions and framework will be revised based on consideration of such comments. The final definitions proposed by the Panel and the Standing Committee on the Scientific Evaluation of Dietary Reference Intakes will be included in the forthcoming Dietary Reference Intakes report on macronutrients, which will include an evaluation of the role of dietary fiber in health.

II.
DEFINITIONS OF DIETARY FIBER

Since the early 1950s, various definitions of dietary fiber have been proposed by different countries and organizations (Table 1). In 1953, Hipsley defined dietary fiber as a term for nondigestible constituents that make up the plant cell wall, encompassing the "unavailable carbohydrate" that had been described much earlier by McCance and Lawrence (1929). This definition was expanded by Trowell (1972) based on: (1) a number of hypotheses relating dietary fiber to health ("dietary fiber hypothesis") including prevention of diverticular disease and colon cancer (Burkitt et al., 1972; Trowell, 1972); (2) a concern for the adverse effects from consuming diets high in refined carbohydrates, termed The Saccharine Disease (Cleave and Campbell, 1966); and (3) the need to replace the term "crude fiber" (Trowell, 1972). Based on the above concerns, dietary fiber was defined as "the skeletal remains of plant cells that are resistant to digestion (hydrolysis) by enzymes of man" (Trowell, 1972).

In 1976, Trowell and colleagues recognized the inadequacy of the 1972 definition because it was not known at the time of the first definition that components of the plant cell other than the cell wall, including mucilages, storage polysaccharides, and algal polysaccharides, were not hydrolyzed by the alimentary enzymes. Therefore, dietary fiber was redefined (Trowell et al., 1976) (Table 1). This definition is synonymous with the term "unavailable carbohydrate", a component of food that was measured by Southgate (1969). Publication of the 1976 definition was the result of interest in the possible health benefits of non-digestible storage polysaccharides, notably guar gum of the cluster bean. This gum was shown to reduce serum cholesterol concentration (Jenkins et al., 1975) and flatten the postprandial glycemia (Gassull et al., 1976).

The 1976 Trowell definition was the basis for the definition set by the Expert Advisory Committee on Dietary Fibre of Health and Welfare Canada (Health and Welfare Canada, 1985) (Table 1). The Health and Welfare Canada definition was initially intended to define dietary fiber with a view to future health claims for fiber. The Committee sought a definition that was broad enough to accommodate the range of dietary fiber values obtained from a number of analytical techniques. The term "endogenous" was added to the definition to emphasize that indigestible materials formed during processing, such as Maillard reaction products or charred carbon, were not considered to be dietary fiber. In addition, water soluble components found in foods, including gums, mucilages, and pectic substances, as well as non-nutritive fiber-associated substances, such as phytates, were intended to be part of dietary fiber.

In 1984, New Zealand Food Regulations defined dietary fiber as the "edible plant material not hydrolysed by the endogenous enzymes of the human digestive tract"; it was to be measured by the first method of analysis (Prosky et al., 1985) accepted by AOAC (AOAC method 985.29).

TABLE 1 Definitions of Dietary Fiber

Reference	Definition
Trowell et al., 1976	Dietary fibre consists of the plant polysaccharides and lignin which are resistant to hydrolysis by digestive enzymes of man.
Health and Welfare Canada, 1985	Dietary fibre is the endogenous components of plant material in the diet which are resistant to digestion by enzymes produced by humans. They are predominantly non-starch polysaccharides and lignin and may include, in addition, associated substances.
U.S. Food and Drug Administration (USFDA), 1987	Dietary fiber is the material isolated by AOAC method 985.29 (see Table 2).
Life Sciences Research Office (LSRO), 1987	Dietary fiber is the endogenous components of plant materials in the diet which are resistant to digestion by enzymes produced by humans.
Health Canada, 1988	A novel fibre source is a food that was manufactured to be a source of dietary fibre, and that (1) had not traditionally been used for human consumption to any significant extent, or (2) had been chemically processed (e.g., oxidized) or physically processed (e.g., finely ground) so as to modify the properties of the fibre, or (3) had been highly concentrated from its plant source.
Anonymous, 1989 (Germany)	Dietary fiber is substances of plant origin, that cannot-be broken down to resorbable components by the body's own enzymes in the small intestine. Included are essentially soluble and insoluble non-starch polysaccharides (cellulose, pectin, hydrocolloids) and lignin and resistant starch. Substances like some sugar substitutes, organic acids, chitin and so on, which either are not or are incompletely absorbed in the small intestine, are not included.
Anonymous, 1992 (Belgium)	Dietary fiber is the components of the foods that are normally not broken down by the body's own enzymes of humans.
Anonymous, 1993 (Italy)	Dietary fiber is the edible substance of vegetable origin which normally is not hydrolyzed by the enzymes secreted by the human digestive system.
FAO/WHO, 1995 (Codex Alimentarius Commission)	Dietary fibre is the edible plant or animal material not hydrolysed by the endogenous enzymes of the human digestive tract as determined by the agreed upon method. (The Codex also approved AOAC methods 985.29 and 991.43 [see Table 2]).

Reference	Definition
Jian-xian, 1995 (China)	Dietary fiber is the sum of food components that are not digested by intestinal enzymes and absorbed into the body.
Denmark, 1995[a]	Dietary fiber is the material isolated by AOAC methods 985.29 and 997.08 (see Table 2).
Ministry of Health and Welfare, 1996 (Japan)	Dietary fiber is the material isolated by the AOAC method 985.29. In addition, non-digestible, low molecular weight carbohydrate determined by high performance liquid chromatography is classified as dietary fiber.
Committee on Medical Aspects of Foods (COMA), 1998 (United Kingdom)	Dietary fibre is non-starch polysaccharide as measured by the Englyst method.
Finland, 1998[a]	Dietary fiber is part of the carbohydrate obtained when using AOAC methods 985.29 and AOAC 997.08 (see Table 2).
Norway, 1998[a]	Dietary fiber is the material isolated by AOAC method 985.29 (see Table 2) and inulin and oligofructose.
Sweden, 1999[a]	Dietary fiber is edible material that cannot be broken down by human endogenous enzymes. Dietary fiber is determined with AOAC method 985.29. In addition, the fructan AOAC method 997.08 may be used (see Table 2).
American Association of Cereal Chemists (AACC), 2000	Dietary fiber is the edible parts of plants or analogous carbohydrates that are resistant to digestion and absorption in the human small intestine with complete or partial fermentation in the large intestine. Dietary fiber includes polysaccharides, oligosaccharides, lignin, and associated plant substances. Dietary fibers promote beneficial physiological effects including laxation, and/or blood cholesterol attenuation, and/or blood glucose attenuation.
Hignett, 2000 (U.K. Food Standards Agency)	Dietary fiber is the material isolated by AOAC methods 985.29 and/or 991.43, combined with 997.08 (see Table 2).
Australia New Zealand Food Authority (ANZFA) (Proposed), 2000	Dietary fibre is that fraction of the edible part of plants or their extracts, or analogous carbohydrates, that are resistant to digestion and absorption in the human small intestine, usually with complete or partial fermentation in the large intestine. The term includes polysaccharides, oligosaccharides (degrees of polymerization >2), and lignins. Dietary fibre promotes one or more of these beneficial physiological effects: laxation, reduction in blood cholesterol, and/or modulation of blood glucose.

[a] N-G Asp, Division of Applied Nutrition, Lund University, personal communication, February 22, 2001.

TABLE 2 Components Measured by the Various Methods of Fiber Analysis

Reference (Method)[a]	Lignin	Nonstarch Polysaccharide	Resistant Starch	Inulin
Asp et al., 1983	Yes	Yes	Some	Some
Craig et al., 2000 (AOAC 2000.11)	No	No	No	No
Englyst and Cummings, 1984 (E-GC)	No	Yes	No	No
Englyst and Hudson, 1987 (E-C)	No	Yes	No	No
Gordon and Ohkuma, in press (AOAC 2001.03)	Yes	Yes	Some	Yes
Hoebregs, 1997 (AOAC 997.08)	No	No	No	Yes
Lee et al., 1992 (AOAC 991.43)	Yes	Yes	Some	Some
Li and Cardozo, 1994 (AOAC 993.21)	Yes	Yes	Some	Some
McCleary et al., 2000 (AOAC 999.03)	No	No	No	Yes
Mongeau and Brassard, 1993 (AOAC 992.16)	Yes	Yes	No	No
Prosky et al., 1985, 1988, 1992, 1994 (AOAC 985.29, 993.19, 991.42)	Yes	Yes	Some	Some
Quigley and Englyst, 1992 (E-HPLC)	No	Yes	No	No
Schweizer and Würsch, 1979	Yes	Yes	Some	Some
Southgate, 1969	Yes	Yes	Some	No
Theander and Åman, 1979	Yes	Yes	Some	No
Theander and Westerlund, 1986	Yes	Yes	Some	No
Uppsala Method of Theander et al., 1995 (AOAC 994.13)	Yes	Yes	Some	No

[a] E-GC = enzymatic-gas chromatographic, E-C = enzymatic-colorimetric, E-HPLC = enzymatic-high performance liquid chromatographic.
[b] Yes, if molecular weight is 12,000 daltons or more.

Oligosaccha-rides	Polydextrose	Resistant Malto-dextrins	Chitin and Chitosan	Chondroitin Sulfate	Noncarbo-hydrate
No	No	No	Some	Some	Some
No	Yes	No	No	No	No
No	No	No	Some	Some	No
No	No	No	Some	Some	No
Yes	Yes	Yes	Some	Some	Some
No	No	No	No	No	No
No	No	No	Some	Some	Some
No	No	No	Some	Some	Some
No	No	No	No	No	No
No	No	No	Some	Some	Some
No	No	No	Some	Some	Some
No	No	No	Some	Some	No
No	No	No	Some	Some	Some
No	No	No	Some	Some	No
No	No	No	Some	Yes[b]	No
No	No	No	Some	Yes[b]	No
No	No	No	Some	Some	No

In 1987, the U.S. Food and Drug Administration (FDA) adopted AOAC method 985.29 for regulatory purposes to identify dietary fiber as a mixture of nonstarch polysaccharides, lignin, and some resistant starch (USFDA, 1987) (Table 1). Related methods that isolated the same components as AOAC method 985.29 were developed independently (AOAC methods 991.42, 991.43, 992.16, 993.19, 993.21, and 994.13; see Table 2) and accepted by AOAC in subsequent years. These methods are also accepted by FDA. The 1976 Trowell definition was the basis for FDA accepting the AOAC methods for isolating dietary fiber. These methods exclude all oligosaccharides (3 to 9 degrees of polymerization) from the definition and include all polysaccharides, lignin, and some of the resistant starch that is resistant to the enzymes (protease, amylase, and amyloglucosidase) used in the AOAC methods. However, FDA did not and still does not have a written definition of dietary fiber for the purposes of food labeling and health claims.

Similar to the United States, there is no official definition of dietary fiber in Japan. A standard method for measuring dietary fiber in Japan is based on AOAC method 985.29 plus a chromatographic method that isolates low molecular weight maltodextrins (Gordon and Ohkuma, in press) (Table 1). Dietary fibers can also be approved in Japan as effective ingredients in foods for specific health use; these include indigestible maltodextrin, hydrolyzed guar gum, chitosan, polydextrose, psyllium, wheat bran, and depolymerized sodium alginate (DeVries, 2001). For many Asian countries, dietary fiber intake tables have been based on AOAC methods 985.29 and 991.43, although the definition used by China since 1995 does not identify a specific method (Jian-xian, 1995) (Table 1).

The Expert Panel on Dietary Fiber of the Life Sciences Research Office (LSRO) proposed a definition of dietary fiber in 1987 similar to the one identified by Health and Welfare Canada in 1985. This definition included nonstarch polysaccharides and lignin and excluded fiber-associated substances found in the plant cell wall such as phytates, cutins, saponins, lectins, proteins, waxes, silicon, and other inorganic components (LSRO, 1987). Other substances not considered to be dietary fiber according to the LSRO definition include indigestible compounds formed during cooking or processing (e.g., resistant starch, Maillard reaction products), oligosaccharides and carbohydrate polymers of less than 50 to 60 degrees of polymerization that are not recovered in dietary fiber analysis, nonplant-derived compounds (e.g., chitin, chitosan), and synthetic carbohydrate polymers.

In 1988, Health Canada published guidelines for novel fiber sources and food products containing them that can be labeled as a source of fiber in addiion to those included in their 1985 definition (Health Canada, 1988) (Table 1). The rationale for these guidelines was that there were safety issues unique to novel sources of fiber, and if a product was represented as containing fiber, it should have the beneficial physiological effects associated with dietary fiber that the public expects. The guidelines indicate that both safety and efficacy of the fiber source have to be established in order for the product to be identified as a source of dietary fiber in Canada, and this has to be done through experiments using human subjects. Three measures of efficacy were identified: (1) laxation, (2) normalization of blood lipid levels, and (3) attenuation of blood glucose responses. Detailed guidelines were later produced for the clinical studies required to assess laxation effects, as this was the physiological function most often used by industry when seeking approval for a novel fiber source (Health Canada, 1997a).

In 1995, a definition for dietary fiber appeared in the Codex Alimentarius Guidelines on Nutrition Labelling (FAO/WHO, 1995) (Table 1). The Codex allows the analytical methods AOAC 985.29 and AOAC 991.43 (Table 2) for measurement of dietary fiber in special foods and infant formula. There have been recent attempts to revise the Codex definition; however, there has not been a consensus on the inclusion of animal and other chemically characterized substances (FAO/WHO, 2000).

Several countries in Europe published definitions for dietary fiber in the late 1980s and early 1990s, including Germany (Anonymous, 1989), Belgium (Anonymous, 1992), and Italy (Anonymous, 1993) (Table 1). For labeling purposes, Denmark, Finland, Norway, and Sweden have defined dietary fiber as edible material that cannot be degraded by human endogenous enzymes, as measured by AOAC method 985.29 (Table 1). The issue regarding inclusion or exclusion of inulin and fructooligosaccharides has been handled somewhat differently by these countries in the absence of European Union regulation. In Denmark and Norway, fructans have been allowed to be included as dietary fiber on the food labels since 1995 and 1998, respectively (i.e., before the approval of AOAC method 997.08). Sweden made a similar decision in 1999, specifying AOAC method 997.08. In 1998, the Food Administration of Finland recommended that inulin and oligofructose be labeled separately and not be included as dietary fiber. In 2001, however, AOAC method 997.08 was added to 985.29 for analysis of dietary fiber, implying that inulin and oligofructose can now be labeled as dietary fiber in the four Nordic countries (N-G Asp, Division of Applied Nutrition, Lund University, personal communication, February 22, 2001).

In 1998, the Committee on Medical Aspects of Food and Nutrition Policy (COMA) of the United Kingdom formally adopted the Englyst nonstarch polysaccharide method for defining dietary fiber (COMA, 1998) (Table 1). In September 2000, the U.K. Food Standards Agency recommended AOAC methods 991.43 and 997.08 (Table 2) to ensure consistent labeling of food products (Hignett, 2000) (Table 1). In November 2000, the U.K. Food Standards Agency acknowledged COMA's definition of dietary fiber as nonstarch polysaccharides yet recognized that the "European rules preclude insistence on a national definition". AOAC method 985.29 and the Englyst method (Englyst and Cummings, 1984) are cur rently accepted by the European Community to measure dietary fiber but there is no clearly written definition of the material that is measured by these methods.

In May 2000, the American Association of Cereal Chemists (AACC) adopted an updated definition of dietary fiber that was developed by a committee appointed to review, and if necessary, update the original AACC definition of dietary fiber (AACC, 2000) (Table 1). This definition is similar to the ANZFA definition. The AACC definition recognizes that the primary characteristics of dietary fiber are resistance to digestion and absorption in the small intestine and fermentation in the large intestine; the rationale for including these characteristics is that it recognizes the key physiological impacts of fiber demonstrated in the past 30 years of research (AACC, 2000).

In November 2000, the recently formed Australia New Zealand Food Authority (ANZFA) concluded that relying on a prescribed analytical method as the sole means of defining dietary fiber for regulatory purposes was unsatisfactory since analytical methods do not take into consideration the physiological impact of new food forms or food ingredients that are part of the diet (ANZFA, 2000). Thus, a definition has been proposed (Table 1) that includes the origin, chemistry, and physiology of dietary fiber, similar to the Codex Alimentarius Guidelines on Nutrition Labelling (FAO/WHO, 1995) and the earlier New Zealand Food Regulations definition (New Zealand, 1984). Furthermore, ANZFA has endorsed the use of AOAC method 985.29 or 991.43, and AOAC methods 997.08 or 999.03, which measure fructans (e.g., inulin) (Table 2).

In conclusion, a variety of definitions for dietary fiber have been promulgated by scientific and regulatory agencies worldwide. Some definitions specifically state a physiological definition of dietary fiber, whereas others rely on more prescribed analytical methods as the sole determinant of dietary fiber. The majority of accepted analytical methods for the measurement of dietary fiber are based on a variety of AOAC accepted methods.

Since many definitions are based on methods to analyze dietary fiber, the evolution of the methodologies to measure fiber were reviewed (see Appendix C). Nonstarch polysaccharides are recovered by all methods designed to measure all components of dietary fiber, and only those methods developed to measure a specific fiber component (e.g., resistant maltodextrins, inulin, polydextrose) do not recover nonstarch polysaccharides (Table 2). Most methods include the non-carbohydrate lignin as a component of dietary fiber. Only the methods of Englyst and the methods developed to measure a specific type of polysaccharide exclude lignin. In addition, the methods of Englyst and of Mongeau and Brassard, which were designed to measure all fiber components, do not include resistant starch as fiber.

Dependence on ethanol precipitation as a means of recovering polysaccharides excludes polydextrose, resistant maltodextrin, and oligosaccharides, and most inulin, which are soluble in ethanol. These saccharides also are lost if ethanol is used at the beginning of an analytical procedure to remove mono- and disaccharides. Measurement of polysaccharides from animal sources (e.g., chitin, chitosan, or chondroitin sulfate) has not been systematically studied, but methods developed to measure total fiber do recover a portion of these types of polysaccharides.

III.

ISSUES IN DEFINING DIETARY FIBER

A careful analysis of the definitions of dietary fiber previously discussed reveals that there are a number of important ways in which one definition differs from another. These differentiating characteristics involve whether the following are included: animal carbohydrates, carbohydrates not recovered by alcohol precipitation, mono- and disaccharides, lignin, and resistant starch, and whether the fiber has to be intact and naturally occurring in food. Resistance to human endogenous digestive enzymes is specified in only some definitions. Some definitions require that a fiber have specific physiological effects, whereas others do not. How each definition has dealt with these issues is summarized in Table 3. Discussion and resolution of each of these differences among existing definitions formed the basis for the proposed definitions.

ANIMAL VERSUS PLANT MATERIAL

Traditionally, the definition of dietary fiber has included only plant substances (Health and Welfare Canada, 1985; LSRO, 1987; Trowell et al., 1976). However, due to the limited methodological approaches that were developed, the accepted methods of measuring dietary fiber do not exclude substances that are not plant based. Thus, compounds like chitosan or glycosaminoglycans (i.e., mucopolysaccharides) derived from animals are included in the fiber analytical values (Table 2). High fiber foods traditionally consumed in a Western diet contain negligible amounts of animal polysaccharides. But, as animal compounds are isolated and marketed as dietary supplements, animal sources that analyze as dietary fiber are becoming more significant. Polysaccharides from animals, yeast, bacteria, and agricultural by-products may all be similar in chemical structure to some components that make up the fiber found in plant foods. Although there has been no thorough evaluation, it can be assumed that animal-derived carbohydrate polymers analyze as dietary fiber by existing fiber methods. Definitions of dietary fiber thus include nondigestible animal carbohydrates (Table 3) in one of two ways: (1) they are part of dietary fiber for all definitions that are based on methods that precipitate polysaccharides with ethanol or measure monosaccharide constituents in the fiber residue, or (2) they are included because the definition does not specify plant components.

As interest in dietary fiber increases, economic incentives drive the development and subsequent marketing of more potential fiber products. Currently in the United States, but not in Canada, if these products assay as fiber by accepted methods, they are included as part of the total fiber content of foods. Furthermore, there are few data from human studies comparing animal-based with plant-based fibers using physiological endpoints. Until such data are available, the role of these animal fiber sources cannot be determined.

CARBOHYDRATES NOT RECOVERED BY ALCOHOL PRECIPITATION

Because many current definitions are based on methods involving ethanol precipitation, oligosaccharides and fructans that are endogenous in foods, but soluble in ethanol, are not analyzed as dietary fiber. Yet endogenous human enzymes do not digest fructans which are found in plants such as chicory, onions, and Jerusalem artichoke; thus they are included in many definitions (Table 3). Quantitation of fructans will be incomplete, even if the constituent monosaccharides of fructans are measured by a procedure that does not include ethanol precipitation, because the fructose component of fructans is labile in many acid hydrolysis procedures used during fiber analysis. Furthermore, fructose can be reduced to sorbitol and mannitol during preparation of derivatives for gas chromatographic analysis.

The oligosaccharides raffinose, stachyose, and verbacose that occur naturally in legumes and a variety of manufactured and enzymatically produced short-chain polysaccharides (e.g., fructooligosaccharides and partially hydrolyzed inulin and guar gum) also do not precipitate in ethanol. Several manufactured carbohydrates, such as methylcellulose, polydextrose, and oligosaccharides, are also resistant to human enzymatic hydrolysis. This would classify them as fiber under may definitions; however, they are not routinely analyzed as dietary fiber because they do not precipitate in ethanol.

No uniform approach has been developed to resolve the issue of fiber carbohydrates that do not precipitate in ethanol, even though many of these naturally occurring, hydrolyzed, or manufactured components are not analyzed as fiber but are considered to be fiber by many definitions. Recent analytical efforts have been directed toward the measurement of a specific carbohydrate or product, such as polydextrose or fructooligosaccharides. This individual approach has resulted in a proliferation of methods, some of which would overlap if applied to a product containing several manufactured or modified carbohydrates.

INCLUSION OR EXCLUSION OF MONO- AND DISACCHARIDES

Typically, mono- and disaccharides have been found to be digestible by humans, and they do not precipitate in ethanol. Thus, no definition, except that used in China, includes these carbohydrates as dietary fiber (Table 3). However, chemical and enzymatic modification of saccharides normally digested and absorbed in humans, such as glucose, or hydrolysis of fiber polysaccharides, such as a gum or inulin, result in mixtures that may contain monosaccharides and disaccharides that are not fully digested and absorbed. Theoretically, monosaccharides, such as arabinose, mannose, xylose, and galacturonic acid, that make up many fiber polysaccharides would be passively absorbed in the human small intestine, although unknown quantities would still reach the large intestine. Without

TABLE 3 Characteristics of Various Dietary Fiber Definitions[a]

Reference	Nondigestible Animal CHOs[b]	CHOs Not Recovered by Alcohol Precipitation[c]	Nondigestible Mono- and Disaccharides
Trowell et al., 1976	No	Not considered	Not considered
Health and Welfare Canada, 1985	No	Not considered	Not considered
U.S. Food and Drug Administration (USFDA), 1987[d]	Yes	Some inulin	No
Life Sciences Research Office (LSRO), 1987	No	No	No
Health Canada, 1988	Yes	Implied[e]	Not considered
Anonymous, 1989 (Germany)	No	No	No
Anonymous, 1992 (Belgium)	Yes	Yes	No
Anonymous, 1993 (Italy)	No	Yes	No
FAO/WHO, 1995 (Codex Alimentarius Commission)[d]	Yes	Some inulin	No
Jian-xian, 1995 (China)	Yes	Yes	Yes
Denmark, 1995[d,f]	Yes	Some inulin	No
Ministry of Health and Welfare, 1996 (Japan)[d]	Yes	Yes	No
Committee on Medical Aspects of Foods (COMA), 1998 (United Kingdom)[d]	Yes	No	No
Finland, 1998[d,f]	Yes	Labeled separately, some inulin	No
Norway, 1998[d,f]	Yes	Inulin and oligofructose	No
Sweden, 1999[d,f]	Yes	Some inulin	No
American Association of Cereal Chemists (AACC), 2000	Yes	Yes	No
Hignett, 2000 (U.K. Food Standards Agency)[c]	Yes	Some inulin	No

Lignin	Resistant Starch	Intact, Naturally Occurring Food Sources Only	Resistant to Human Enzymes	Specifies Physiological Effect
Yes	Not considered	Not specifically listed	Yes	No
Yes	Not specifically listed	Yes	Yes	No
Yes	Some	No	No	No
Yes	No	Yes	Yes	No
Implied	Implied	No	Implied	No
Yes	Yes	No	Yes	No
Yes	Yes	No	Yes	No
Yes	Yes	No	Yes	No
Yes	Some	No	Yes	No
Yes	Yes	No	Yes	No
Yes	Some	No	No	No
Yes	Some	No	No	No
No	No	No	No	No
Yes	Some	Implied	Implied	No
Yes	Some	No	No	No
Yes	Some	No	No	No
Yes	Yes	No	Yes	Yes
Yes	Some	No	No	No

Reference	Nondigestible Animal CHOs[b]	CHOs Not Recovered by Alcohol Precipitation[c]	Nondigestible Mono- and Disaccharides
Australia New Zealand Food Authority (ANZFA) (Proposed), 2000	Yes	Yes	No
Institute of Medicine (Proposed), 2001			
Dietary Fiber	No	Yes	No
Added Fiber	Yes	Yes	Yes

[a] All definitions are assumed to include nonstarch polysaccharides.
[b] CHO = carbohydrate.
[c] Includes inulin, oligosaccharides (3–10 degrees of polymerization), fructans, polydextrose, methylcellulose, resistant maltodextrins and other related compounds.

specific disaccharidases, it is unlikely that disaccharides of these fiber-derived sugars or chemically modified disaccharides of glucose could be digested in the human small intestine. Because these mono- and disaccharides are nondigestible or poorly absorbed in the human small intestine, they could be classified as fiber.

The issue of including special mono- and disaccharides as dietary fiber has not been resolved. Methodological differentiation of digestible and nondigestible mono- and disaccharides will be cumbersome and complex to accomplish. Furthermore, these materials physiologically act as classic osmotically active agents in the gut, much in the same way that sugar alcohols do, and this response has not previously been considered a mechanism of action for dietary fiber.

LIGNIN

Although not a carbohydrate, lignin, a phenylpropane polymer, is typically included in the definition of dietary fiber (Table 3). Lignin is covalently bound to fibrous polysaccharides (Jung and Fahey, 1983) and has a heterogeneous composition ranging from one or two units to many phenyl propanes that are cyclically linked. These two characteristics have probably formed the basis for defining lignin as dietary fiber. Furthermore, although lignin is present in the human food supply in very small amounts, animal research with high fiber feeds has shown that lignin affects the physiological effects of dietary fiber. For example, lignin hinders fermentation of fiber polysaccharides in ruminants (Titgemeyer et al., 1991).

Lignin	Resistant Starch	Intact, Naturally Occurring Food Sources Only	Resistant to Human Enzymes	Specifies Physiological Effect
Yes	Yes	No	Yes	Yes
Yes	Some	Yes	Yes	No
Yes	Yes	No	Yes	Yes

[d] Method-based definition.
[e] Implied means not stated but inferred.
[f] N-G Asp, Division of Applied Nutrition, Lund University, personal communication, February 22, 2001.

RESISTANT STARCH

The early definitions for dietary fiber did not consider resistant starch as its presence was not yet recognized (Table 3). Only the definitions proposed by LSRO (1987) and COMA (1998) specifically exclude resistant starch. The 1998 COMA definition is based on the Englyst method of analysis, which removes all starch from the fiber residue by solubilization with dimethyl sulfoxide. Some definitions, such as those of Germany and AACC, include resistant starch by specifically listing it; for others, such as those used in Belgium, Italy, and China, the wording of the definition indicates that resistant starch is part of fiber. Most other definitions, including the definition from the U.K. Food Standards Agency (Hignett, 2000), incorporate variable amounts of resistant starch as dietary fiber because they are based on AOAC procedures that do not analyze a portion of starch during fiber analysis (AOAC 991.43 and 997.08).

Depending on one's chosen diet, naturally occurring and manufactured resistant starch, as well as that produced during normal processing of foods for human consumption, could make a significant contribution to daily fiber intake. Legumes are the single largest source of naturally occurring resistant starch (Marlett and Longacre, 1996). In addition, green bananas (Englyst and Cummings, 1986) and cooled, cooked potatoes (Englyst and Cummings, 1987) can provide a significant amount of resistant starch. Resistant starch resulting from normal processing of a foodstuff is a more modest contributor to a typical daily intake. Starches specifically manufactured to be resistant to endogenous human digestion are a rapidly growing segment of commercially available resistant starches. Physiological effects and analysis of resistant starch are being intensively studied (Asp, 1997). Several issues remain to be addressed in these re search areas, particularly for the emerging manufactured resistant starches. The development of an analytical method that reflects the extent of their digestion in vivo in the human stomach and small intestine is also needed.

INTACT AND NATURALLY OCCURRING IN FOOD

The dietary fiber hypotheses of Burkitt and colleagues (1972) and Trowell (1972) were based on populations consuming unrefined diets that were high in dietary fiber and slowly digested carbohydrates. Fiber-rich foods, however, contain micronutrients and many other biologically active compounds that have distinct physiological and biochemical effects in humans. Furthermore, fiber integrated into plant cellular structure is released or becomes a viable force in the gastrointestinal tract only as digestible nutrients are hydrolyzed during digestion. These two features of fiber-rich foods are undoubtedly contributors to some of the health benefits usually attributed to dietary fiber.

As interest has increased in fiber, manufacturers have isolated dietary fiber from a wide range of carbohydrate sources to be added to foods. Many of these isolated materials are used as food additives based on functional properties such as thickening or fat reduction. As enzymatic and other technologies evolve, many types of polysaccharides will continue to be designed and manufactured using plant and animal synthetic enzymes. Examples in this category include modified cellulose in which the hydroxyl groups on the glucose residues have been substituted to varying degrees with alkyl groups such as methyl and propyl; fructooligosaccharides manufactured from sucrose; and polydextrose synthesized from glucose. In some instances, fibers isolated from plants or manufactured chemically or synthetically have demonstrated more powerful beneficial physiological effects than a food source of the fiber polysaccharide; in other instances, isolation from the plant matrix decreases physiological benefit.

Specificity of the various dietary fiber definitions with respect to non- or undigestibilty of the material varies among definitions (Table 3). Twelve of the current definitions specify or imply resistance to human enzymes, and seven do not. Some experts believe that resistance to human endogenous enzymatic digestion is a necessary component of the definition to ensure that degradation (i.e., fermentation) occurs in the human large intestine through the metabolism of fiber by the resident microflora.

REQUIREMENT THAT A FIBER HAVE SPECIFIC HEALTH BENEFITS

Two recent promulgated definitions (AACC, 2000; ANZFA, 2000) have specific health benefits necessary for a material to be labeled or considered to be dietary fiber (Table 3). However, origins of the current interest in dietary fiber came from observations that populations that consumed diets high in dietary fiber had reduced incidence of several chronic diseases common in Western populations. Correlational studies compared the incidence of heart disease, colon cancer, diverticular disease, diabetes, and other diseases with estimates of crude fiber in the diet of rural African populations and the United States (Burkitt et al., 1974). Since the health benefits of dietary fiber will be extensively reviewed in the upcoming report on Dietary Reference Intakes for macronutrients, only those health benefits previously considered and relevant to the fiber definition are briefly discussed here.

Colonic Health

One of the oldest recognized effects of dietary fiber is modulation of intestinal function. Dietary fiber alters water content, viscosity, and microbial mass of intestinal contents, resulting in changes in the rate and ease of passage through the intestine. The result of increased fiber includes reduced transit time, increased fecal weight, and improved laxation (Birkett et al., 1997), which, along with dilution of lumenal contents, have been proposed to reduce colon cancer risk (Trock et al., 1990). The accompanying reduction in intracolonic pressure may lower diverticular disease risk (Brodribb and Humphreys, 1976). By comparing effects of many different fiber sources, it has become apparent that those fibers that are slowly, incompletely, or not fermented significantly increase stool output; these fibers usually analyze as insoluble fibers and contrast with soluble fibers, most of which are rapidly fermented.

Correlational epidemiological evidence suggests a relationship between dietary fiber intake and colon cancer incidence (Trock et al., 1990), but more refined case control studies have observed a less consistent effect (Lanza, 1990). Furthermore, epidemiological observations suggest that formation of adenomatous polyps, a precancerous colonic lesion, is related to dietary fiber intake (Giovannucci et al., 1992), but colon cancer incidence is not (Giovannucci et al., 1994). Two recently published intervention trials, of 3 years duration, found no effect of fiber on the recurrence of adenomatous polyps in subjects given a wheat bran fiber supplement (Alberts et al., 2000) or in subjects who consumed a diet low in fat and high in fruits, vegetables, and fiber (Schatzkin et al., 2000). Wheat bran has been shown to reduce concentrations of fecal bile acids (Alberts et al., 1996), which have been implicated as carcinogenic promoters or cocarcinogens. In summary, the body of evidence indicates that slowly digested or nonfermentable fiber sources promote laxation, but evidence is insufficient to determine if decreased colon cancer risk is a beneficial effect of fiber. The complex etiology of colon cancer and the significant genetic involvement make the design of appropriate intervention trials very difficult except through the use of alternate end points, which has thus far been unsuccessful.

Breast Cancer

Some evidence has also accumulated suggesting a relationship between dietary fiber consumption and breast cancer risk (Gerber, 1998). However, this relationship is less consistent than that of fiber and colon cancer. Although intervention trials suggest an ability of fiber to reduce blood estrogen concentration, which is a risk factor for the development of breast cancer (Rose et al., 1991), data are not sufficient to suggest that high fiber diets lower breast cancer risk.

Cardiovascular Disease

A relatively large body of experimental data (Anderson et al., 2000; Olson et al., 1997; Ripsin et al., 1992) support a blood cholesterol-lowering effect of viscous dietary fibers that usually analyze as soluble fibers, and epidemiological evidence supports the relationship between increased intake of foods high in fiber and decreased risk of cardiovascular disease (Rimm et al., 1996; Wolk et al., 1999). In contrast, intervention with wheat bran had no significant effect on blood cholesterol concentrations (Anderson et al., 1991), failing to support an epidemiological benefit on cardiovascular disease incidence.

Using blood cholesterol concentrations as a marker for cardiovascular disease, certain fibers have beneficial physiological effects by lowering blood cholesterol, probably by modifying sterol balance (Anderson et al., 1984; Everson et al., 1992; Marlett et al., 1994). Experiments using viscous isolated polysaccharides (e.g., pectin, psyllium, guar gum) as a fiber source have demonstrated that many retain this hypocholesterolemic characteristic in the isolated form (Brown et al., 1999). Some evidence also suggests an inverse relationship between fiber and hypertension, another risk factor for cardiovascular disease (Ascherio et al., 1992, 1996). It is unclear whether fiber itself or substances associated with fiberrich foods, such as phytochemicals and minerals, may be the important factors in the effects observed in these epidemiological studies.

Diabetes

The role of high fiber diets in reducing risk for Type 2 diabetes mellitus and for treatment of both forms of diabetes also relates to viscosity. Viscous fibers from food reduce glycemic response better than sources rich in nonviscous fibers (e.g., cellulose and lignin) (Wolever and Jenkins, 1993), and increase insulin sensitivity (Fukagawa et al., 1990). Increased viscosity results in slower stomach emptying, slower rate of absorption, and changes in the composition of colonic microbial flora (Roberfroid, 1993). Epidemiological studies have found that high glycemic load and low cereal fiber consumption is positively correlated with risk of Type 2 diabetes (Salmerón et al., 1997a, 1997b). In addition, blood glucose concentrations are reduced and exogenous insulin needs are lower when individuals with Type 2 diabetes consume higher fiber diets (Anderson and Ward, 1979). The beneficial physiological effects of viscous fibers on blood glucose concentrations have been consistently demonstrated for over 25 years and are supported by more mechanistic studies.

Hydrolysis reduces viscosity of guar gum and mixed linkage β-glucan (Jenkins et al., 1978; Wood et al., 1994) and hydrolyzed versions are now available because the lower viscosity may increase potential for additional food uses. However, what data exist on the physiological differences seen when polymeric chain length and viscosity are reduced suggest that the glycemic and cholesterol-lowering effects of fiber may be reduced or lost (Favier et al., 1997; Jenkins et al., 1978; Lund et al., 1989; Wood et al., 1994). Therefore, the advantages of improved palatability and ease of use must be weighed against potential loss of physiological effect for fibers that have a shorter chain length and reduced viscosity.

Obesity

A fiber-rich diet has been suggested to be an important factor in weight maintenance and the treatment of obesity (Appleby et al., 1998; Burley et al., 1993; Miller et al., 1994), although the significant changes in upper gastrointestinal tract function are difficult to consistently measure. Diets high in fiber are associated with slower stomach emptying, which induces a short-term increase in satiety (Roberfroid, 1993). This may modulate caloric intake and the rate of nutrient absorption. In addition, the reduced caloric density of diets rich in fiber has been suggested to be an asset in weight maintenance. Diets higher in fiber are just one aspect of the treatment of obesity, and at this time, measurable effects attributable solely to fiber are insufficient to designate fiber as a beneficial physiological effector of body weight.

Other Roles in Health

There are several other potential beneficial effects of fiber and fiber-like materials for which additional data are needed before the benefits can be substantiated. For example, some preliminary observational evidence suggests fiber may protect against duodenal ulcers (Aldoori et al., 1997) and gastric cardia cancer (Terry et al., 2001). Animal experiments have suggested a role of various fibers on intestinal immune function (Field et al., 1999; Lim et al., 1997), although human studies are lacking. As a result of fiber serving as substrate for bacteria in the large intestine, changes in the spectrum and mass of bacteria in the intestine have been a topic of discussion for some time (Roberfroid, 1993). As these changes are more thoroughly understood, the use of fibers to modify fecal and colonic bacteria, much like the suggested use of probiotics, may be possible.

IV.
PROPOSED DEFINITION OF DIETARY FIBER

The Panel on the Definition of Dietary Fiber proposes two definitions to encompass current and future nondigestible carbohydrates in the food supply that are considered to be meaningful subdivisions of the potential substances that could be included:

1. *Dietary Fiber* consists of nondigestible carbohydrates and lignin that are intrinsic and intact in plants.
2. *Added Fiber* consists of isolated, nondigestible carbohydrates that have beneficial physiological effects in humans.
   Total Fiber is the sum of *Dietary Fiber* and *Added Fiber*.

This two-prong approach to define edible, nondigestible carbohydrates recognizes the diversity of carbohydrates in the human food supply that are not digested: plant cell wall and storage carbohydrates that predominate in foods, carbohydrates contributed by animal foods, and isolated and low molecular weight carbohydrates that occur naturally or have been synthesized or otherwise manufactured. These definitions recognize a continuum of carbohydrates and allow for flexibility to incorporate new fiber sources developed in the future following demonstration of beneficial physiological effects in humans.

DISTINGUISHING FEATURES

Dietary Fiber consists of nondigestible food plant carbohydrates and lignin in which the plant matrix is largely intact. Nondigestible means that the material is not digested and absorbed in the human small intestine. Nondigestible plant carbohydrates in foods are usually a mixture of polysaccharides that are integral components of the plant cell wall or intercellular structure (see Table 3). This definition recognizes that the three-dimensional plant matrix is responsible for some of the physicochemical properties attributed to *Dietary Fiber*. Fractions of plant foods are considered *Dietary Fiber* if the plant cells and their three-dimensional interrelationships remain largely intact. Thus, mechanical treatment would still result in intact fiber. Another distinguishing feature of *Dietary Fiber* sources is that they contain other macronutrients (e.g., digestible carbohydrate and protein) normally found in foods. For example, cereal brans, which are obtained by grinding, are anatomical layers of the grain consisting of intact cells and substantial amounts of starch and protein; they would be categorized as *Dietary Fiber* sources. Resistant starch that is naturally occurring and inherent in a food or created during normal processing of a food, as is the case for flaked corn cereal, would be categorized as *Dietary Fiber*. Examples of oligosaccharides that fall under the category of *Dietary Fiber* are those that are normally constituents of a *Dietary Fiber* source, such as raffinose, stachyose, and verba cose in legumes, and the low molecular weight fructans in foods, such as Jerusalem artichoke and onions.

Added Fiber consists of isolated or extracted nondigestible carbohydrates that have beneficial physiological effects in humans. *Added Fibers* may be isolated or extracted using chemical, enzymatic, or aqueous steps. Synthetically manufactured or naturally occurring isolated oligosaccharides and manufactured resistant starch are included in this definition. Also included are those naturally occurring polysaccharides or oligosaccharides usually extracted from their plant source that have been modified, for example to a shorter polymer length or to a different molecular arrangement. Although it has been inadequately studied, animal-derived carbohydrates such as connective tissue are generally regarded as nondigestible. The fact that animal-derived carbohydrates are not of plant origin forms the basis for including animal-derived, nondigestible carbohydrates in the *Added Fiber* category. Isolated, manufactured, or synthetic oligosaccharides of three or more degrees of polymerization are considered to be *Added Fiber*. Nondigestible monosaccharides, disaccharides, and sugar alcohols are not considered *Added Fiber* because they fall under "carbohydrates" on the food label.

RATIONALE FOR DEFINITIONS

Nondigestible carbohydrates are frequently isolated to concentrate a desirable attribute of the mixture from which it was extracted. Distinguishing a category of *Added Fiber* allows for the desirable characteristics of such components to be highlighted. In the relatively near future, plant and animal synthetic enzymes may be produced as recombinant proteins, which in turn may be used in the manufacture of fiber-like materials. The definition will allow for the inclusion of these materials and will provide a viable avenue to synthesize specific oligosaccharides and polysaccharides that are part of plant and animal tissues.

Three established physiological effects of *Added Fibers* are recognized at this time as beneficial to human health. These are attenuation of postprandial blood glucose concentrations, attenuation of blood cholesterol concentrations, and improved laxation. Rapidly changing lumenal fluid balance resulting from large amounts of nondigestible mono- and disaccharides or low molecular weight oligosaccharides, such as what occurs when sugar alcohols are consumed, is not considered a mechanism of laxation for *Added Fibers.*

Nondigestible carbohydrates may influence specific aspects of immune function, particularly since the small intestine embodies quantitatively the largest proportion of immune tissue in mammals (Kelly and Coutts, 2000; McKay and Perdue, 1993). Furthermore, nearly all fibers are fermented to some extent, producing short-chain fatty acids for which a variety of physiologic roles are being identified (Bugaut and Bentejac, 1993; Fleming and Yeo, 1990; Mortensen and Clausen, 1996). However, insufficient data and a lack of consistency in available experimental results limit recognition of some beneficial physiological effects related to immune function at this time. The two-pronged approach to defining fiber, however, allows for future addition of these and other beneficial physiological effects as they are identified and characterized with some certainty.

In summary, one definition has been proposed for *Dietary Fiber* because many other substances in high fiber foods, including a variety of vitamins and minerals, often have made it difficult to demonstrate a significant health benefit specifically attributable to the fiber in foods. Thus, it is difficult to separate out the effect of fiber per se from the high fiber food. Attempts have been made to do this, particularly in epidemiological studies, by controlling for other substances in those foods, but these attempts were not always successful. The advantage, then, of adding isolated nondigestible carbohydrates as a fiber source to a food is that one may be able to draw conclusions about *Added Fiber* itself with regard to its physiological role rather than the vehicle in which it is found. The proposed definitions do not preclude research directed towards the health benefits of *Dietary Fiber* in foods, but it is not necessary to demonstrate a physiological effect in order for a food fiber to be listed as *Dietary Fiber*.

Two important aspects of the recommended definitions are that some fibers are *Added Fibers* and that a substance is required to demonstrate a beneficial physiological effect to be classified as *Added Fiber*. Research has shown that extraction or isolation of a polysaccharide, usually through chemical, enzymatic, or aqueous means, can either enhance its health benefit (usually because it is a more concentrated source) or diminish the beneficial effect. These recommendations should be helpful in evaluating diet and disease relationship studies as one will be able to classify fiber-like components as *Added Fibers* due to their documented health benefits. Although databases are not currently constructed to delineate potential beneficial effects of specific fibers, there is no reason that this could not be accomplished in the future.

INCLUSION OF LIGNIN AS DIETARY FIBER

It is recognized that lignin consists of phenolic compounds and not carbohydrates. Although lignin is present in the North American food supply in only small amounts, it is included as *Dietary Fiber* for two reasons: it is covalently bound to fiber polysaccharides, and its presence alters the physiological effects of the fiber. For example, fermentability of fiber polysaccharides is reduced by lignin (Jung, 1989; Titgemeyer et al., 1991). Definitions of dietary fiber promulgated by Health and Welfare Canada, Germany, and AACC, as well as the definition proposed by ANZFA, specifically include lignin. Lignin is the only fiber-associated substance included in the definition of *Dietary Fiber* and is only included when it is part of the intact plant matrix.

EXCLUSION OF SPECIFIC PHYSIOLOGICAL EFFECTS

Specific physiological effects are not part of the definitions because new beneficial effects of nondigestible carbohydrates will continue to be discovered. Furthermore, the aim of this activity was to promulgate definitions that have overall long-term applicability. Thus specific physiological benefits are not included because such a definition would become quickly outdated as new health effects become established. It is anticipated that acceptable physiological benefits will be identified during implementation of the proposed definitions.

PHASING OUT THE TERMS SOLUBLE AND INSOLUBLE DIETARY FIBER

Physiological effects of some ingested *Dietary Fibers* and some *Added Fibers* include attenuation of postprandial blood glucose concentration and blood cholesterol concentration and improved laxation. Available data suggest that the addition of fiber sources that are viscous are capable of altering blood glucose and cholesterol concentrations (Anderson et al., 1999; Jenkins et al., 1978, 2000). Fiber sources that are slowly, incompletely, or essentially not fermented in the large intestine provide bulk and therefore optimize laxation (Birkett et al., 1997; Cummings, 1997). These two physicochemical properties, viscosity and fermentability, are recommended as meaningful alternative characteristics for the terms soluble and insoluble fiber to distinguish *Dietary Fibers* and *Added Fibers* that modulate gastric and small bowel function from those that provide substantial stool bulk. It is recommended that the terms soluble and insoluble fiber be phased out and replaced with the appropriate physicochemical property as the characterization of the properties of various fibers becomes standardized.

V.
IMPACT OF THE DEFINITIONS OF DIETARY FIBER AND UNRESOLVED ISSUES

Adoption of these proposed definitions will have significant impact in a variety of areas. In particular, major developments and modifications will be needed in the area of fiber analysis, and additional research into physiological actions of many fibers will be necessary. The results of these new efforts will be reflected in food composition databases and on the nutrient label, and resources and collaborative efforts will be needed from the food industry, research and analytical scientists, and governments.

However, these definitions are a true improvement over existing definitions because they begin to recognize fiber as a nutrient with demonstrable health effects and lessen the emphasis on fiber as a constituent of food requiring quantitation; this improvement warrants the adaptations that will have to occur. Anticipated changes and unresolved issues are the focus of this section.

IMPACT ON ANALYTICAL METHODOLOGY

The proposed definitions, based on health benefits and physiological considerations rather than on analytical methods, will undoubtedly have major impact on the analysis of fiber. Analytical methods are needed that will fit with the definitions, not the reverse. This approach to defining fiber recognizes dietary fiber as a nutrient, rather than merely as an analytically measured food constituent.

The Panel was not charged with proposing methods for fiber analysis that would be consistent with the new definitions. It was, however, charged with proposing definition(s) that would take into consideration possibilities for analysis. It is anticipated that analysis for the proposed fiber definitions will be approached from two directions concurrently. One will explore development of new methods of characterization and analysis, and the other will involve modification of existing methods to accommodate the new definitions. It is also recognized that the ideal analytical approach would be to have methods for *Dietary Fiber* and for *Added Fiber*, with the sum of the two results being *Total Fiber*. Current methodology, including approaches for specific *Added Fibers,* are reviewed in Appendix C, with overall approaches outlined below.

Several changes to current methods are needed to obtain values for *Dietary Fiber. Dietary Fiber* now includes all naturally occurring resistant starch, not just that portion measured by current enzymatic-gravimetric methods. Thus, methodological modifications are needed that extract all resistant starch from fiber and then measure this fiber. Complete extraction of resistant starch from fiber has been accomplished by some analytical methods, and it is likely that complete starch removal can be accomplished by incorporating either additional enzymes that hydrolyze starch or the solvent dimethyl sulfoxide into the current procedures. Several methods for specifically measuring resistant starch are now under evaluation, and some approaches are likely to measure that fraction resistant to the actions of the human stomach and small intestine and therefore, be suitable for application to all foods. Consideration should be given to methods that not only determine resistant starch, but also measure digestible or total starch in the same assay so that a portion of the total starch is not recovered in more than one starch fraction. Naturally occurring oligosaccharides inherent in foods containing *Dietary Fiber* need to be captured during analysis. Since most oligosaccharides are not recovered by ethanol precipitation, it may be necessary to recover them from the ethanol soluble fraction on the basis of molecular weight by chromatography or dialysis.

Current fiber analysis methods recover animal polysaccharides as dietary fiber. Thus, for those foods containing any animal carbohydrates, methods for their analysis are needed so they can be subtracted from the *Dietary Fiber* value. A general method applicable to all animal carbohydrates that would distinguish them from plant carbohydrates is difficult to envision. For those *Dietary Fibers* containing animal carbohydrates, however, it may be possible to use specific enzymatic steps to hydrolyze glycosaminoglycans (i.e., mucopolysaccharides), glycoproteins, or other carbohydrates in cartilage for subsequent quantitation. Perhaps an amount of animal-derived carbohydrates in *Dietary Fiber* could be defined below which the animal carbohydrate could be disregarded. For example, if 10 percent or less of the *Dietary Fiber* were from animals, it would not have to be determined and subtracted from the *Dietary Fiber*.

Some possible approaches for analyzing for *Dietary Fiber* that utilize unmodified current methods of analysis include:

    a.   Using gravimetric methods:

1. gravimetric methods (AOAC methods 985.29, 991.43, 992.16, 993.21)
2. subtract resistant starch
3. subtract nondigestible, animal-derived carbohydrate
4. add naturally occurring resistant starch
5. add naturally occurring oligosaccharides

    b.   Using the method of Theander:

1. method of Theander
2. subtract resistant starch
3. subtract nondigestible, animal-derived carbohydrate
4. add naturally occurring resistant starch
5. add naturally occurring oligosaccharides

c. Using the appropriate method of Englyst:

1. method of Englyst (colorimetric, GC, or HPLC)
2. subtract nondigestible, animal-derived carbohydrate
3. add lignin
4. add naturally occurring resistant starch
5. add naturally occurring oligosaccharides

The fibers that are included in the definition of *Added Fiber* could be analyzed using methods for each specific compound that have been or could be developed, generally using GC or HPLC for quantitation after the *Added Fiber* has been isolated, typically by chromatography or dialysis. In some instances, *Added Fiber* could be determined enzymatically, for example, as mixed linkage β-glucan is now (McCleary and Codd, 1991). Existing analytical methods for *Total Fiber* would be suitable for those *Added Fibers* that are quantitatively recovered by the method.

The possibility that more than one *Added Fiber* might be in a food product also needs to be addressed. In this case, different *Added Fibers* may be distinguished by their specific method of analysis. Alternately, they may be distinguishable on the basis of monosaccharide composition or by enzymatic hydrolysis. For example, mixed linkage β-glucan could be measured enzymatically, as it currently is. Monosaccharide composition data would be available only if the fiber was isolated from the food matrix, acid hydrolyzed to yield the constituent carbohydrates, and those monosaccharides individually quantitated by GC or HPLC. A knowledge of the monosaccharide composition of the individual *Added Fiber* is required for this approach. *Total Fiber* analysis, analysis for individual *Added Fibers* by specific methods, and formulation or recipe information may be needed for analysis of complex mixtures of *Added Fibers*.

The most challenging analytical issue is the analysis of food products for fiber when they contain both *Dietary Fiber* and *Added Fiber*. It is likely that a combination of existing and new methods, similar to what has been illustrated above, will be needed to effectively separate and quantitate these two types of fiber when they occur in the same food vehicle. A measurement of *Total Fiber* is still possible, but formulation information and analyses for specific *Added Fibers* by appropriate methods may need to be combined with analytical data to distinguish *Dietary Fiber* and *Added Fiber*. However, it may be more practical to determine *Total Fiber* using either current methods or modifications of current methods for *Total Fiber* and to follow up with continued development of methods to determine *Added Fibers*.

While development of new methods requires dedicated input from industry, academia, and government, the exploration of using more modern analytical approaches for the analysis of *Dietary Fiber* and *Added Fiber* is encouraged. Methods already exist that specifically and accurately measure fiber-derived polysaccharides by determining the amounts of their constituent neutral monosaccharides by GC or HPLC and the acidic polymers that comprise pectin by a colorimetric assay. The incorporation of a step using dimethyl sulfoxide, as is done in the Englyst methods, could extract all starch from fiber. An additional analysis to measure naturally occurring resistant starch would be needed for foods. For foods containing oligosaccharides or other ethanol soluble carbohydrates, an additional step would be needed whereby these carbohydrates would be recovered from the ethanol on the basis of molecular weight, using column chromatography or dialysis; they could be combined with the fiber-derived carbohydrates for quantitative analysis. Conceivably, a multi-part procedure could be developed and approved, and only those steps relevant to the fiber source being analyzed would need to be performed.

IMPACT ON RECOMMENDED LEVELS OF INTAKE

It is not anticipated that these definitions would significantly impact recommended levels of intake. However, information on both *Dietary Fiber* and *Added Fiber* would more clearly delineate the source of fiber and the potential health benefits. Although these two categories of fiber would be listed separately, the *Total Fiber* recommendation would reflect the sum of the two. The rationale for summing the two is that naturally occurring *Dietary Fiber* has known, although difficult to delineate, health benefits, and substances presented as *Added Fiber* could not be included on the label without a demonstrated beneficial physiological effect. Thus, *Added Fiber* should contribute to human health just as *Dietary Fiber* does and should count toward the total recommended level of intake. It is also possible that where the physiological benefits of each type of fiber, *Dietary Fiber or Added Fiber,* are well characterized, separate recommendations for intake could be constructed.

A separate issue involves potential Tolerable Upper Intake Levels (UL) for fiber. The possible adverse effects of fiber, including *Dietary Fiber* and *Added Fiber,* will be reviewed in the upcoming report that will provide Dietary Reference Intakes (DRIs) for macronutrients. It may be possible to concentrate large amounts of *Added Fiber* in foods, beverages, and supplements. Since the potential adverse health effects *of Added Fiber* are not completely known, they should be evaluated on a case-by-case basis. In addition, projections regarding the potential contribution of *Added Fiber* to daily *Total Fiber* intake at anticipated patterns of food consumption would be informative.

IMPACT ON FOOD COMPOSITION DATABASES

More information on food carbohydrates will be required with these new definitions, much in the way that more detailed information on protein (i.e., amino acids) and fat (i.e., fatty acids) has been incorporated into food tables.

Values for *Dietary Fiber* and *Added Fiber* would be listed under *Total Fiber*. Each of these categories could be further divided and contain data on constituents. Constituents under *Added Fiber* could include isolated, modified, and synthesized carbohydrates, such as mixed linkage β-glucans, pectins, celluloses, some resistant starches, gums, and oligosaccharides. Constituents under *Dietary Fiber* could include intrinsic and intact celluloses, hemicelluloses, pectins, lignin, resistant starches, and mixed linkage β-glucans. Given the difficulty in developing methods that provide physiologically relevant values, no data for the amounts of soluble and insoluble fiber would appear in the food composition tables. At least three values would be listed in the food composition database: *Total Fiber*, *Dietary Fiber*, and *Added Fiber*. As noted earlier, current methods may need to be modified and new methods will need to be developed to provide these compositional data.

IMPACT ON DIETARY FIBER RESEARCH

Although many aspects of the health benefits of fiber and fiber-containing foods remain poorly understood and in need of investigation, four areas of research are particularly relevant to the proposed definitions. First, research to identify and meaningfully and reproducibly assess established physiological effects of fiber on laxation and blood glucose and cholesterol concentrations, or other possible beneficial effects, is needed for a material to be classified as *Added Fiber*. Second, research is needed to develop and evaluate appropriate methods to measure viscosity and fermentability in such a way that the in vitro data obtained can be related to in vivo action. Third, there is a need to continue research that identifies and characterizes new and emerging physiological effects of existing fibers. Finally, discovery and characterization of new materials that could be classified as *Added Fiber* should continue.

Although the proposed definitions do not outline the nature and extent of demonstrating a beneficial health effect for *Added Fiber*, it is anticipated that research designs used to characterize the established physiological effects on laxation and blood glucose and cholesterol concentrations can form the basis for developing standard protocols and criteria to determine whether an *Added Fiber* demonstrates one of these beneficial physiological effects. In addition, the possibility of using analytically determined viscosity and fermentability as part of the evaluation process needs to be explored. Using all of these avenues for evaluation will encourage the development of new *Added Fibers* and broaden the diversity of materials with special health benefits.

The intention of replacing the concept of soluble and insoluble fibers with viscous and incompletely fermented fibers is to bring into use analytically obtained characteristics that have physiological relevance. Appropriate standards and controls need to be identified, as do conditions of experimentation, such as time, temperature, and concentration. Also, procedures need to be applied to the fiber and not the food, as food products may be made viscous through other ingredients and processing.

Similarly, an in vitro system that accurately reflects the rate and extent of fermentation of a material in the human large intestine will need to be devised and evaluated for application to *Added Fibers*. The relevance of a proposed analytical approach to in vivo behavior will need to be determined in a variety of circumstances. The analytical procedure will also need to be evaluated for ruggedness, relevance to various in vivo situations, and analytical accuracy and precision.

Several areas are emerging as potential physiological effects of *Dietary Fiber* and *Added Fiber*. More research could be conducted on the potential use of *Dietary Fiber* and *Added Fiber* in weight control, as certain fibers reduce food intake and possibly the amount of metabolizable energy available. In addition, there are alleged physiological effects of dietary fibers where too few data now exist to demonstrate a role conclusively, but which will have great relevance should the link between fiber and physiological effect be clearly established. These include the effects of fiber on colonic ecology, gut hormones, and the immune system.

In addition, the relationship between the biochemical characteristics of *Dietary Fibers* (e.g., monosaccharide composition, biologically active plant cell wall fragments [arabinoxylans], and linkages between carbohydrate moieties and other cell wall components like lignin) and physiological events need further clarity and are deserving of enhanced research activity. In the case of oligosaccharides, their role as *Dietary* or *Added Fiber* versus serving as osmotically active agents in the gut needs to be clarified. Acute and rapid changes in colonic lumenal fluid, such as what is produced by sugar alcohols, has not traditionally been a mechanism of action for fiber. The proposed definitions include nondigestible carbohydrates of low molecular weight (oligosaccharides of three or more sugar residues), and research is needed to determine the relative benefits and risks of relatively large amounts of low molecular weight fiber oligosaccharides.

Accurate, repeatable measures of colonic health must be established. For instance, little is known about the metabolic activities of the microbes in the human large intestine that may be exposed to atypical substrates or, in certain instances, subjected to starvation conditions. Indeed, data collected using molecular-based systems for identification of microbes may result in a reevaluation of what is presently accepted about the microbial ecology of the gut, most of which has been determined by plating techniques. What are the rates and extents of substrate fermentation that optimize conditions in the lower gut vis-a-vis health status? Further, the long-term consequences of crowding out certain strains of bacteria by feeding particular dietary fibers are unknown. Questions such as these must be answered to improve understanding of the effect of fiber on colonic health status.

Despite the established fact that dietary fiber is considered a healthful part of the diet, dietary fiber intakes in the United States are only about half of recommended levels (Alaimo et al. 1994), and surveys indicate that the majority of Canadians are not concerned with the amount of fiber in their diet (Federal, Provincial and Territorial Advisory Committee on Population Health, 1999). Chronic inadequate fiber intakes give manufacturers reason to supplement foods with fiber and to market fiber supplements. In the United States, consumers recognize dietary fiber as a positive component of the food supply, and its inclusion on a food label is thought to have significant impact. In particular, concentrating a desirable material as an *Added Fiber* will allow the health benefits of its presence in the product to be emphasized.

Because *Dietary Fiber* is the fiber that occurs naturally in plant foods, labeling for fruits, vegetables, whole grains, legumes, and nuts will continue unchanged under the proposed definition in both the United States and Canada. This could lead to increased utilization of natural plant foods in food products, which is in keeping with recent dietary recommendations to consume more grains, especially whole grain, fruits, and vegetables (Health Canada, 1997b; USDA/DHHS, 2000). Since the proposed definition of *Dietary Fiber* includes naturally occurring resistant starch, starchy foods such as legumes or pasta may also be utilized to a greater extent in food products to provide *Dietary Fiber*.

Currently in the United States, to claim that a product contains dietary fiber requires that the fiber content be based on accepted AOAC methods. Inulin, polydextrose, resistant starch, and some other isolated carbohydrates are not assayed by these methods. Therefore, under current regulations, these substances do not qualify as dietary fiber. However, many manufacturers have conducted clinical studies that show their products have positive physiological properties similar to those of accepted fiber sources; many of these substances now may be eligible to qualify as *Added Fiber* under the new definitions. For new and untested materials, demonstration of a beneficial physiological effect will be necessary for the substance to qualify as an *Added Fiber*. Research has supported three health benefits (attenuation of blood glucose and cholesterol concentrations and improved laxation) *of Added Fiber*. Although protocols to demonstrate efficacy of a new product are not specified as part of the proposed definition, it is recognized that food manufacturers will need information on the characteristics and types of studies required to demonstrate beneficial physiological effects. It is also recognized that the food industry will have to allocate resources to substantiate the beneficial health effect of an *Added Fiber* product.

IMPACT ON NUTRITION LABELING

Adoption of the proposed definitions will have a positive, informative impact on nutrition labeling. The current system of labeling for dietary fiber— dietary fiber, insoluble and/or soluble—will be replaced by two values: *Dietary Fiber* and *Added Fiber*. After an education process, consumers will learn that both *Dietary Fiber* and *Added Fiber* are considered to play a role in health. *Dietary Fiber* will include plant foods in which the fiber is relatively intact and nutrients other than fiber that are present and may contribute significantly to the attributed overall health effects. *Added Fiber* will contain only those fibers shown to have positive health benefits. It is assumed that the food industry will promote the health benefits of their *Added Fibers*, and therefore, consumers will be able to anticipate the types of beneficial effects that may occur if they consume foods containing these *Added Fibers*. In the future it is anticipated that the specific types of *Added Fibers* will be part of the food label, thus providing the consumer and health professional with additional information. *Total Fiber* will be the sum of *Dietary Fiber* and *Added Fiber*, so if the consumer wants to know the total amount of fiber per serving this value will provide that information. Since it is recommended that the current designations "soluble" and "insoluble" dietary fiber be eliminated from the label, their removal will provide space for the inclusion of *Dietary Fiber* and *Added Fiber*.

As discussed earlier, a separate issue regarding nutrition labeling centers on accurate analytical verification of the division of *Total Fiber* into *Dietary Fiber* and *Added Fiber*. In addition, dietary fiber is currently assigned an energy value of 0 kcal/g if it is insoluble and 4 kcal/g if it is soluble. Although not a task of this report, the complexity of assigning these somewhat arbitrary energy values to dietary fiber is discussed in detail in Appendix D.

VI. REFERENCES

Åkerberg AKE, Liljeberg HGM, Granfeldt YE, Drews AW, Björck IME. 1998. An in vitro method, based on chewing, to predict resistant starch content in foods allows parallel determination of potentially available starch and dietary fiber. *J Nutr* 128: 651–660.

Alaimo K, McDowell MA, Briefel RR, Bischof AM, Caughman CR, Loria CM, Johnson CL. 1994. Dietary intake of vitamins, minerals, and fiber of persons ages 2 months and over in the United States: Third National Health and Nutrition Examination Survey, Phase 1, 1988–91. Advance Data from Vital and Health Statistics, No. 258. Hyattsville, MD: National Center for Health Statistics.

Alberts DS, Ritenbaugh C, Story JA, Aickin M, Rees-McGee S, Buller MK, Atwood J, Phelps J, Ramanujam PS, Bellapravalu S, Patel J, Bettinger L, Clark L. 1996. Randomized, double-blinded, placebo-controlled study of effect of wheat bran fiber and calcium on fecal bile acids in patients with resected adenomatous colon polyps. *J Natl Cancer Inst* 88: 81–92.

Alberts DS, Martínez ME, Roe DJ, Guillén-Rodríguez JM, Marshall JR, van Leeuwen JB, Reid ME, Ritenbaugh C, Vargas PA, Bhattacharyya AB, Earnest DL, Sampliner RE. 2000. Lack of effect of a high-fiber cereal supplement on the recurrence of colorectal adenomas. *N Engl J Med* 342: 1156–1162.

Aldoori WH, Giovannucci EL, Stampfer MJ, Rimm EB, Wing AL, Willett WC. 1997. Prospective study of diet and the risk of duodenal ulcer in men. *Am J Epidemiol* 145: 42–50.

Anderson JW, Ward K. 1979. High-carbohydrate, high-fiber diets for insulin-treated men with diabetes mellitus. *Am J Clin Nutr* 32: 2312–2321.

Anderson JW, Story L, Sieling B, Chen W-JL, Petro MS, Story JA. 1984. Hypercholesterolemic effects of oat-bran or bean intake for hypercholesterolemic men. *Am J Clin Nutr* 40: 1146–1155.

Anderson JW, Gilinsky NH, Deakins DA, Smith SF, O'Neal DS, Dillon DW, Oeltgen PR. 1991. Lipid responses of hypercholesterolemic men to oat-bran and wheat-bran intake. *Am J Clin Nutr* 54: 678–683.

Anderson JW, Allgood LD, Turner J, Oeltgen PR, Daggy BP. 1999. Effects of psyllium on glucose and serum lipid responses in men with type 2 diabetes and hypercholesterolemia. *Am J Clin Nutr* 70: 466–473.

Anderson JW, Allgood LD, Lawrence A, Altringer LA, Jerdack GR, Hengehold DA, Morel JG. 2000. Cholesterol-lowering effects of psyllium intake adjunctive to diet therapy in men and women with hypercholesterolemia: Meta-analysis of 8 controlled trials. *Am J Clin Nutr* 71: 472–479.

Anonymous. 1989. GDch Stellungnahme der Untergruppe "Ballaststoffe" der Arbeitsgruppe "Freagen der Emahrung" der Fachgruppe "Lebensmittelchemie und gerichtliche Chemie" in der GDCh". *Lebensmittelchemie und Gerichtliche Chemie* 43: 113–117.

Anonymous. 1992. Belgian Food Law, KB 8/1/1992.

Anonymous. 1993. Italian Food Law, DL 16/2/1993.

Anonymous. 2000. AACC holds midyear meeting. *Cereal Foods World* 45: 327.

ANZFA (Australia New Zealand Food Authority). 2000. *Notice of a Proposed Change to Food Regulation and Further Invitation for Submissions. Application 227. Inulin and Fructooligosaccharides as Dietary Fibre*. Canberry: ANZFA.

VI. REFERENCES

AOAC (Association of Official Analytical Chemists). 1995. *Official Methods of Analysis of the Association of Official Analystical Chemists*, 16th edition. Horowitz W, ed. Washington, DC: AOAC. Pp. 18–19.

Appleby PN, Thorogood M, Mann JI, Key TJ. 1998. Low body mass index in non-meat eaters: The possible roles of animal fat, dietary fibre and alcohol. *Int J Obes* 22: 454–460.

Argenzio RA, Miller N, von Engelhardt W. 1975. Effect of volatile fatty acids on water and ion absorption from the goat colon. *Am J Physiol* 229: 997–1002.

Ascherio A, Rimm EB, Giovannucci EL, Colditz GA, Rosner B, Willett WC, Sacks F, Stampfer MJ. 1992. A prospective study of nutritional factors and hypertension among US men. *Circulation* 86: 1475–1484.

Ascherio A, Hennekens C, Willett WC, Sacks F, Rosner B, Manson J, Witteman J, Stampfer MJ. 1996. Prospective study of nutritional factors, blood pressure, and hypertension among US women. *Hypertension* 27: 1065–1072.

Asp N-G. 1997. Resistant starch—An update on its physiological effects. In: Kritchevsky D, Bonfield C, eds. *Dietary Fiber in Health and Disease*. New York: Plenum Press. Pp. 201–210.

Asp N-G, Johansson C-G. 1981. Techniques for measuring dietary fiber: Principal aims of methods and a comparison of results obtained by different techniques. In: James WPT, Theander O, eds. *The Analysis of Dietary Fiber in Food*. New York: Marcel Dekker. Pp. 173–189.

Asp N-G, Johansson C-G, Hallmer H, Siljeström M. 1983. Rapid enzymatic assay of insoluble and soluble dietary fiber. *J Agric Food Chem* 31: 476–482.

Asp N-G, van Amelsvoort JMM, Hautvast JGAJ. 1996. Nutritional implications of resistant starch. *Nutr Res Rev* 9: 1–31.

Birkett AM, Jones GP, de Silva AM, Young GP, Muir JG. 1997. Dietary intake and faecal excretion of carbohydrate by Australians: Importance of achieving stool weights greater than 150 g to improve faecal markers relevant to colon cancer risk. *Eur J Clin Nutr* 51: 625–632.

Björck I, Nyman M, Pedersen B, Siljeström M, Asp N-G, Eggum BO. 1986. On the digestibility of starch in wheat bread—Studies in vitro and in vivo. *J Cereal Sci* 4: 1–11.

Brodribb AJM, Humphreys DM. 1976. Diverticular disease: Three studies. Part II—Treatment with bran. *Br Med J* 1: 425–428.

Brown L, Rosner B, Willett WC, Sacks FM. 1999. Cholesterol-lowering effects of dietary fiber: A meta-analysis. *Am J Clin Nutr* 69: 30–42.

Bugaut M, Bentejac M. 1993. Biological effects of short-chain fatty acids in nonruminant mammals. *Ann Rev Nutr* 13: 217–241.

Burkitt DP, Walker ARP, Painter NS. 1972. Effect of dietary fibre on stools and transittimes, and its role in the causation of disease. *Lancet* 2: 1408–1412.

Burkitt DP, Walker ARP, Painter NS. 1974. Dietary fiber and disease. *J Am Med Assoc* 229: 1068–1074.

Burley VJ, Paul AW, Blundell JE. 1993. Sustained post-ingestive action of dietary fibre: Effects of a sugar-beet-fibre-supplemented breakfast on satiety. *J Hum Nutr Diet* 6: 253–260.

Champ M. 1992. Determination of resistant starch in foods and food products: Interlaboratory study. *Eur J Clin Nutr* 46: S51–S62.

Champ M, Kozlowski F, Lecannu G. 2001. In-vivo and in-vitro methods for resistant starch measurement. In: McCleary BV, Prosky L, eds. *Advanced Dietary Fibre Technology*. Oxford: Blackwell Science. Pp. 106–119.

Cleave TL, Campbell GD. 1966. *Diabetes, Coronary Thrombosis, and the Saccharine Disease*. Bristol, England: John Wright and Sons.

VI. REFERENCES

COMA (Committee on Medical Aspects of Food and Nutrition Policy). 1998. Committee news. *Food Safety Information Bulletin*, No. 97. Aberdeen, Scotland: Food Standards Agency, MAFF, Department of Health.

Craig SAS, Holden JF, Khaled MY. 2000. Determination of polydextrose as dietary fiber in foods. *J AOAC Int* 83: 1006–1012.

Cummings, JH. 1997. Bowel habit and constipation. In: Institut Danone, ed. *The Large Intestine in Nutrition and Disease*. Bruxelles: Institut Danone. Pp. 87–101.

de Slegte J. In press. Determination of trans-galactooliogsaccharides in selected food products by ion-exchange chromatography: Collaborative study. *J AOAC Int.*

DeVries JW. 2001. Analytical issues regarding the regulatory aspects of dietary fibre nutrition labelling. In: McCleary BV, Prosky L, eds. *Advanced Dietary Fibre Technology*. Oxford: Blackwell Science. Pp. 123–138.

Englyst HN, Cummings JH. 1984. Simplified method for the measurement of total non-starch polysaccharides by gas-liquid chromatography of constituent sugars as alditol acetates. *Analyst* 109: 937–942.

Englyst HN, Cummings JH. 1986. Digestion of the carbohydrates of banana (*Musa paradisiaca sapientum*) in the human small intestine. *Am J Clin Nutr* 44: 42–50.

Englyst HN, Cummings JH. 1987. Digestion of polysaccharides of potato in the small intestine of man. *Am J Clin Nutr* 45: 423–431.

Englyst HN, Hudson GJ. 1987. Colorimetric method for routine measurement of dietary fibre as non-starch polysaccharides. A comparison with gas-liquid chromatography. *Food Chem* 24: 63–76.

Englyst H, Wiggins HS, Cummings JH. 1982. Determination of the non-starch polysaccharides in plant foods by gas-liquid chromatography of constituent sugars as alditol acetates. *Analyst* 107: 307–318.

Englyst HN, Kingman SM, Cummings JH. 1992a. Classification and measurement of nutritionally important starch fractions. *Eur J Clin Nutr* 46: S33–S50.

Englyst HN, Quigley ME, Hudson GJ, Cummings JH. 1992b. Determination of dietary fibre as non-starch polysaccharides by gas-liquid chromatography. *Analyst* 117: 1707–1714.

Englyst HN, Quigley ME, Hudson GJ. 1994. Determination of dietary fibre as non-starch polysaccharides with gas-liquid chromatographic, high-performance liquid chromatographic or spectrophotometric measurement of constituent sugars. *Analyst* 119: 1497–1509.

Everson GT, Daggy BP, McKinley C, Story JA. 1992. Effects of psyllium hydrophilic mucilloid on LDL-cholesterol and bile acid synthesis in hypercholesterolemic men. *J Lipid Res* 33: 1183–1192.

Fahey GC, Grieshop CM. 2000. *Analysis of the Net Energy Value of Two Soluble Fibers*. Bethesda, MD: Life Sciences Research Office, American Society of Nutritional Sciences. Pp. 1–28.

FAO/WHO (Food and Agriculture Organization of the United Nations/World Health Organization). 1995. *Guidelines for Nutrition Labelling*. Codex Alimentarius, Volume 1A, General Requirements. Rome: FAO.

FAO/WHO (Food and Agriculture Organization of the United Nations/World Health Organization). 2000. *Progress Report on Dietary Fibre*. Codex Committee on Nutrition and Foods for Special Dietary Uses, Codex Alimentarius Commission. CX/NFSDU 00/3-Add.2. Rome: FAO.

Favier ML, Bost PE, Guittard C, Demigne C, Remesy C. 1997. The cholesterol-lowering effect of guar gum is not the result of a simple diversion of bile acids toward fecal excretion. *Lipids* 32: 953–959.

VI. REFERENCES

Federal, Provincial and Territorial Advisory Committee on Population Health. 1999. *Statistical Report on the Health of Canadians*. Ottawa: Health Canada.

Field CJ, McBurney MI, Massimino S, Hayek MG, Sunvold GD. 1999. The fermentable fiber content of the diet alters the function and composition of canine gut associated lymphoid tissue. *Vet Immunol Immunopathol* 72: 325–341.

Fleming SE, Yeo S. 1990. Production and absorption of short-chain fatty acids. In: Kritchevsky D, Bonfleld C, Anderson JW, eds. *Dietary Fiber: Chemistry, Physiology, and Health Effects*. New York: Plenum Press. Pp. 301–315.

Fukagawa NK, Anderson JW, Hageman G, Young VR, Minaker KL. 1990. Highcarbohydrate, high-fiber diets increase peripheral insulin sensitivity in healthy young and old adults. *Am J Clin Nutr* 52: 524–528.

Furda I. 1977. Fractionation and examination of biopolymers from dietary fiber. *Cereal Foods World* 22: 252–254.

Gassull MA, Goff DV, Haisman P, Hockaday TDR, Jenkins DJA, Jones K, Leeds AR, Wolever TMS. 1976. The effect of unavailable carbohydrate gelling agents in reducing the postprandial glycaemia in normal volunteers and diabetics. *J Physiol* 259: 52P–53P.

Gerber, M. 1998. Fibre and breast cancer. *Eur J Cancer Prev* 7: S63–S67.

Giovannucci E, Stampfer MJ, Colditz G, Rimm EB, Willett, WC. 1992. Relationship of diet to risk of colorectal adenoma in men. *J Natl Cancer Inst* 84: 91–98.

Giovannucci E, Rimm EB, Stampfer MJ, Colditz GA, Ascherio A, Willett WC. 1994. Intake of fat, meat, and fiber in relation to risk of colon cancer in men. *Cancer Res* 54: 2390–2397.

Goering HK, Van Soest PJ. 1970. *Forage Fiber Analyses (Apparatus, Reagents, Procedures, and Some Applications)*. Agriculture Handbook No. 379. Washington, DC: US Department of Agriculture.

Goñi I, García-Diz L, Mañas E, Saura-Calixto F. 1996. Analysis of resistant starch: A method for foods and food products. *Food Chem* 56: 445–449.

Gordon DT, Ohkuma, K. In press. Determination of resistant maltodextrin and total dietary fiber in selected foods by ion-exchange chromatography: Collaborative study. *J AOAC Int*.

Gove PB, ed. 1967. *Webster's Third International Dictionary*. Springfield, MA: G&C Merriam Company.

Health and Welfare Canada. 1985. *Report of the Expert Advisory Committee on Dietary Fibre*. Ottawa: Supply and Services Canada.

Health Canada. 1988. *Guideline Concerning the Safety and Physiological Effects of Novel Fibre Sources and Food Products Containing Them*. Ottawa: Food Directorate, Health Protection Branch, Health Canada.

Health Canada. 1997a. Appendix 2. Guideline for planning and statistical review of clinical laxation studies for dietary fibre. In: *Guideline Concerning the Safety and Physiological Effects of Novel Fibre Sources and Food Products Containing Them*. Ottawa: Food Directorate, Health Protection Branch, Health Canada.

Health Canada. 1997b. *Canada's Food Guide to Healthy Eating for People Four Years and Over*. Ottawa: Minister of Public Works and Government Services Canada.

Hellendoom EW, Noordhoff MG, Slagman J. 1975. Enzymatic determination of the indigestible residue (dietary fibre) content of human food. *J Sci Food Agric* 26: 1461–1468.

Henneberg W, Stohmann F. 1860. Beitrage zur Begrundung einer rationellen Futterung der Wiederkauer, I. Braunschweig.

VI. REFERENCES

Hignett R. 2000. *Letter to All Interested Parties. Nutrition Labelling of Dietary Fibre*. [Online]. Available: http://foodstandards.gov.uk/farm_fork/nutfibre.htm [accessed March 14, 2001].

Hipsley EH. 1953. Dietary "fibre" and pregnancy toxaemia. *Br Med J* 2: 420–422.

Hoebregs H. 1997. Fructans in foods and food products, ion-exchange chromatographic method: Collaborative study. *J AOAC Int* 80: 1029–1037.

Høverstad T, Fausa O, Bjørneklett A, Bøhmer T. 1984. Short-chain fatty acids in the normal human feces. *Scand J Gastroenterol* 19: 375–381.

Hungate RE. 1966. *The Rumen and its Microbes*. New York: Academic Press.

Jenkins DJA, Newton C, Leeds AR, Cummings JH. 1975. Effect of pectin, guar gum, and wheat fibre on serum cholesterol. *Lancet* 1: 1116–1117.

Jenkins DJA, Wolever IMS, Leeds AR, Gassull MA, Haisman P, Dilawari J, Goff DV, Metz GL, Alberti KGMM. 1978. Dietary fibres, fibre analogues, and glucose tolerance: Importance of viscosity. *Br Med J* 1: 1392–1394.

Jenkins DJA, Kendall CWC, Axelsen M, Augustin LSA, Vuksan V. 2000. Viscous and nonviscous fibres, nonabsorbable and low glycaemic index carbohydrates, bloodlipids and coronary heart disease. *Curr Opin Lipidol* 11: 49–56.

Jian-xian Z. 1995. Active polysaccharides. In: *Functional Foods*. Beijing: China Light Industry Publishing House. P. 10.

Jung HG. 1989. Forage lignins and their effects on fiber digestibility. *Agron J* 81: 33–38.

Jung HG, Fahey GC. 1983. Nutritional implications of phenolic monomers and lignin: A review. *J Anim Sci* 57: 206–219.

Kelly D, Coutts AG. 2000. Early nutrition and the development of immune function in the neonate. *Proc Nutr Soc* 59: 177–185.

Lanza E. 1990. National Cancer Institute Satellite Symposium on Fiber and Colon Cancer. In: Kritchevsky D, Bonfield C, Anderson JW, eds. *Dietary Fiber: Chemistry, Physiology, and Health Effects*. New York: Plenum Press. Pp. 383–387.

Lee SC, Prosky L, DeVries JW. 1992. Determination of total, soluble, and insoluble die-tary fiber in foods—Enymatic-gravimetric method, MES-TRIS buffer: Collaborative study. *J AOAC Int* 75: 395–416.

Li BW, Cardozo MS. 1994. Determination of total dietary fiber in foods and products with little or no starch, nonenzymatic-gravimetric method: Collaborative study. *J AOAC Int* 77: 687–689.

Lim BO, Yamada K, Nonaka M, Kuramoto Y, Hung P, Sugano M. 1997. Dietary fibers modulate indices of intestinal immune function in rats. *J Nutr* 127: 663–667.

Livesey, G. 1990. Energy values of unavailable carbohydrate and diets: An inquiry and analysis. *Am J Clin Nutr* 51: 617–637.

LSRO (Life Sciences Research Office). 1987. *Physiological Effects and Health Consequences of Dietary Fiber*. Bethesda, MD: LSRO.

Lund EK, Gee JM, Brown JC, Wood PJ, Johnson IT. 1989. Effect of oat gum on the physical properties of the gastrointestinal contents and on the uptake of D-galactose and cholesterol by rat small intestine in vitro. *Br J Nutr* 62: 91–101.

Marlett JA, Longacre MJ. 1996. Comparison of in vitro and in vivo measures of resistant starch in selected grain products. *Cereal Chem* 73: 63–68.

Marlett JA, Hosig KB, Vollendorf NW, Shinnick FL, Haack VS, Story JA. 1994. Mechanism of serum cholesterol reduction by oat bran. *Hepatology* 20: 1450–1457.

McCance RA, Lawrence RD. 1929. *The Carbohydrate Content of Foods*. London: HMSO.

McCleary BV. 200la. Measurement of dietary fibre components: The importance of enzyme purity, activity and specificity. In: McCleary BV, Prosky L, eds. *Advanced Dietary Fibre Technology*. Oxford: Blackwell Science Press. Pp. 89–105.

VI. REFERENCES

McCleary BV. 2001b. Two issues in dietary fibre measurement. *Cereal Foods World* 46: 164–166.

McCleary BV, Blakeney AB. 1999. Measurement of inulin and oligofructan. *Cereal Food World* 44: 398–406.

McCleary BV, Codd R. 1991. Measurement of (1-3)(1-4)-β-D-glucan in barley and oats. A streamlined enzymatic procedure. *J Sci Food Agric* 55: 303–312.

McCleary BV, Murphy A, Mugford DC. 2000. Measurement of total fructan in foods by enzymatic/ spectrophotometric method: Collaborative study. *J AOAC Int* 83: 356–364.

McKay DM, Perdue MH. 1993. Intestinal epithelial function: The case for immunophysiological regulation. Cells and mediators (first of two parts). *Dig Dis Sci* 38: 1377–1387.

Miller TL, Wolin MJ.1979. Fermentations by saccharolytic intestinal bacteria. *Am J Clin Nutr* 32: 164–172.

Miller WC, Niederpruem MG, Wallace JP, Lindeman AK. 1994. Dietary fat, sugar, and fiber predict body fat content. *J Am Diet Assoc* 94: 612–615.

Ministry of Health and Welfare. 1996. Regarding the Analytical Methods for Nutritional Components in Connection with Introduction of the Standards for Nutrition Labeling. Notification by the Environmental Health Bureau, Eishin No. 47.

Mongeau R, Brassard R. 1993. Enzymatic-gravimetric determination in foods of dietary fiber as sum of insoluble and soluble fiber fractions: Summary of collaborative study. *J AOAC Int* 76: 923–925.

Mortensen PB, Clausen MR. 1996. Short-chain fatty acids in the human colon: Relation to gastrointestinal health and disease. *Scand J Gastroenterol Suppl* 31: 132–148.

Muir JG, O'Dea K. 1992. Measurement of resistant starch: Factors affecting the amount of starch escaping digestion in vitro. *Am J Clin Nutr* 56: 123–127.

New Zealand. 1984. *Food Regulations 1984*. Wellington, New Zealand: Government Printer.

Olson BH, Anderson SM, Becker MP, Anderson JW, Hunninghake DB, Jenkins DJA, LaRosa JC, Rippe JM, Roberts DCK, Stoy DB, Summerbell CD, Truswell AS, Wolever TMS, Morris DH, Fulgoni VL. 1997. Psyllium-enriched cereals lower blood total cholesterol and LDL cholesterol, but not HDL cholesterol, in hypercholesterolemic adults: Results of a meta-analysis. *J Nutr* 127: 1973–1980.

Paul AA, Southgate DAT. 1978. *McCance and Widdowson's 'The Composition of Foods'*, 4th edition. London: HMSO.

Prosky L, Asp N-G, Furda I, DeVries JW, Schweizer TF, Harland BF. 1985. Determination of total dietary fiber in foods and food products: Collaborative study. *J Assoc Off Anal Chem* 68: 677–679.

Prosky L, Asp N-G, Schweizer TF, DeVries JW, Furda I. 1988. Determination of insoluble, soluble, and total dietary fiber in foods and food products: Interlaboratory study. *J Assoc Off Anal Chem* 71: 1017–1023.

Prosky L, Asp N-G, Schweizer TF, DeVries JW, Furda I. 1992. Determination of insoluble and soluble dietary fiber in foods and food products: Collaborative study. *J AOAC Int* 75: 360–367.

Prosky L, Asp N-G, Schweizer TF, DeVries JW, Furda I, Lee SC. 1994. Determination of soluble dietary fiber in foods and food products: Collaborative study. *J AOAC Int* 77: 690–694.

Quigley ME, Englyst HN. 1992. Determination of neutral sugars and hexosamines by high-performance liquid chromatography with pulsed amperometric detection. *Analyst* 117: 1715–1718.

VI. REFERENCES

Quigley ME, Englyst HN. 1994. Determination of the uronic acid constituents of non-starch polysaccharides by high-performance liquid chromatography with pulsed amperometric detection. *Analyst* 119: 1511–1518.

Rimm EB, Ascherio A, Giovannucci E, Spiegelman D, Stampfer MJ, Willett WC. 1996. Vegetable, fruit, and cereal fiber intake and risk of coronary heart disease among men. *J Am Med Assoc* 275: 447–451.

Ripsin CM, Keenan JM, Jacobs DR, Elmer PJ, Welch RR, Van Horn L, Liu K, Turnbull WH, Thye FW, Kestin M, Hegsted M, Davidson DM, Davidson MH, Dugan LD, Demark-Wahnefried W, Beling S. 1992. Oat products and lipid lowering: A meta-analysis. *J Am Med Assoc* 267: 3317–3325.

Roberfroid M. 1993. Dietary fiber, inulin, and oligofructose: A review comparing their physiological effects. *Crit Rev Food Sci Nutr* 33: 103–148.

Rose DP, Goldman M, Connolly JM, Strong LE. 1991. High-fiber diet reduces serum estrogen concentrations in premenopausal women. *Am J Clin Nutr* 54: 520–525.

Salmerón J, Ascherio A, Rimm EB, Colditz GA, Spiegelman D, Jenkins DJ, Stampfer MJ, Wing AL, Willett WC. 1997a. Dietary fiber, glycemic load, and risk of NIDDM in men. *Diabetes Care* 20: 545–550.

Salmerón J, Manson JE, Stampfer MJ, Colditz GA, Wing AL, Willett WC. 1997b. Dietary fiber, glycemic load, and risk of non-insulin-dependent diabetes mellitus in women. *J Am Med Assoc* 277: 472–477.

Sandford PA, Baird J. 1983. Industrial utilization of polysaccharides. In: Aspinall GO, ed. *The Polysaccharides*, Vol 2. New York: Academic Press. pp. 411–490.

Schatzkin A, Lanza E, Corle D, Lance P, Iber F, Caan B, Shike M, Weissfeld J, Burt R, Cooper MR, Kikendall JW, Cahill J. 2000. Lack of effect of a low-fat, high-fiber diet on the recurrence of colorectal adenomas. *N Engl J Med* 342: 1149–1155.

Schweizer TF, Würsch P. 1979. Analysis of dietary fibre. *J Sci Food Agric* 30: 613–619.

Shinnick FL, Longacre MJ, Ink SL, Marlett JA. 1988. Oat fiber: Composition versus physiological function in rats. *J Nutr* 118: 144–151.

Smith T, Brown JC, Livesey G. 1998. Energy balance and thermogenesis in rats consuming nonstarch polysaccharides of various fermentabilities. *Am J Clin Nutr* 68: 802–819.

Southgate DAT. 1969. Determination of carbohydrates in foods. II. Unavailable carbohydrates. *J Sci Food Agric* 20: 331–335.

Southgate DAT. 1981. Use of the Southgate method for unavailable carbohydrates in the measurement of dietary fiber. In: James WPT, Theander O, eds. *The Analysis of Dietary Fiber in Food*. New York: Marcel Dekker. Pp. 1–19.

Terry P, Lagergren J, Ye W, Wolk A, Nyren O. 2001. Inverse association between intake of cereal fiber and risk of gastric cardia cancer. *Gastroenterology* 120: 387–391.

Theander O, Åman P. 1979. Studies on dietary fibres. 1. Analysis and chemical characterization of water-soluble and water-insoluble dietary fibres. *Swedish J Agric Res* 9: 97–106.

Theander O, Westerlund E. 1986. Determination of individual components of dietary fiber. In: Spiller GA, ed. *CRC Handbook of Dietary Fiber in Human Nutrition*. Boca Raton, FL: CRC Press. Pp. 57–75.

Theander O, Åman P, Westerlund E, Graham H. 1994. Enzymatic/chemical analysis of dietary fiber. *J AOAC Int* 77: 703–709.

Theander O, Åman P, Westerlund E, Andersson R, Pettersson D. 1995. Total dietary fiber determined as neutral sugar residues, uronic acid residues, and Klason lignin (the Uppsala method): Collaborative study. *J AOAC Int* 78: 1030–1044.

VI. REFERENCES

Titgemeyer EC, Cameron MG, Bourquin LD, Fahey GC. 1991. Digestion of cell wall components by dairy heifers fed diets based on alfalfa and chemically treated oat hulls. *J Dairy Sci* 74: 1026–1037.

Trock B, Lanza E, Greenwald P. 1990. Dietary fiber, vegetables, and colon cancer: Critical review and meta-analyses of the epidemiologic evidence. *J Natl Cancer Inst* 82: 650–661.

Trowell H. 1972. Crude fibre, dietary fibre and atherosclerosis. *Atherosclerosis* 16: 138–140.

Trowell HC, Southgate DAT, Wolever TMS, Leeds AR, Gassull MA, Jenkins DJA. 1976. Dietary fibre redefined. *Lancet* 1: 967.

USDA/DHHS (U.S. Department of Agriculture/Department of Health and Human Services). 2000. *Nutrition and Your Health: Dietary Guidelines for Americans*. Home and Garden Bulletin No. 232. Washington, DC: Government Printing Office.

USFDA (U.S. Food and Drug Administration). 1987. Nutrition labeling of food; calorie content. *Federal Register* 52: 28590–28691.

Van Soest PJ. 1963. Use of detergents in the analysis of fibrous feeds. II. A rapid method for the determination of fiber and lignin. *J Assoc Off Agric Chem* 46: 829–835.

Van Soest P, Wine RH. 1967. Use of detergents in the analysis of fibrous feeds. IV. Determination of plant cell wall constituents. *J Assoc Off Agric Chem* 50: 50–55.

Watt BK. 1976. *Composition of Foods: Raw, Processed, Prepared*. Agriculture Handbook No. 8. Washington, DC: Agricultural Research Service, U.S. Department of Agriculture.

Williams RD, Olmsted WH. 1935. A biochemical method for determining indigestible residue (crude fiber) in feces: Lignin, cellulose, non-water-soluble hemicelluloses. *J Biol Chem* 108: 653–666.

Wolever TMS, Jenkins DJA. 1993. Effect of dietary fiber and foods on carbohydrate metabolism. In: Spiller GA, ed. *CRC Handbook of Dietary Fiber in Human Nutrition*. Boca Raton, FL: CRC Press. Pp. 111–152.

Wolk A, Manson JE, Stampfer MJ, Colditz GA, Hu FB, Speizer FE, Hennekens CH, Willett WC. 1999. Long-term intake of dietary fiber and decreased risk of coronary heart disease among women. *J Am Med Assoc* 281: 1998–2004.

Wood PJ, Braaten JT, Scott FW, Riedel KD, Wolynetz MS, Collins MW. 1994. Effect of dose and modification of viscous properties of oat gum on plasma glucose and insulin following an oral glucose load. *Br J Nutr* 72: 731–743.

VI. REFERENCES

Appendix A
Acknowledgments

The Panel on the Definition of Dietary Fiber, the Standing Committee on the Scientific Evaluation of Dietary Reference Intakes, and the Food and Nutrition Board (FNB) staff are grateful for the time and effort of the many contributors to the report and the workshop and meetings leading up to the report. Through openly sharing their considerable expertise and different outlooks, these individuals and organizations brought clarity and focus to the challenging task of developing a definition for fiber. The list below mentions those individuals who we worked closely with, but many others also deserve our heartfelt thanks. Those individuals, whose names we do not know, made important contributions to the report by offering suggestions and opinions at the many professional meetings and workshops the Panel members attended. The Panel and Committee members, as well as the FNB staff thank the following named (as well as unnamed) individuals and organizations:

INDIVIDUALS

Nils-Georg Asp	Mark Izzo
Michael Auerbach	David Kritchevsky
Jonathan DeVries	Betty Li
Victor Fulgoni	Michael McBurney
Daniel Gallaher	Barry McCleary
Dennis Gordon	

ORGANIZATIONS

American Society for Nutritional Sciences
Calorie Control Council
Federal Advisory Steering Committee for Dietary Reference Intakes
Health Canada
International Life Sciences Institute, N.A.

Appendix B

Glossary

Cellulose. Cellulose, a polysaccharide consisting of linear β-(1,4)-linked glucopyranoside units, is the main structural component of plant cell walls. Humans lack digestive enzymes to cleave β-(1,4) linkages and thus cannot absorb glucose from cellulose.

Chitin and Chitosan. Chitin is a polysaccharide analogous in chemical structure to cellulose except that the repeating unit is a (1,4)-linked N-acetyl-D-glucosamine, a compound consisting of glucose derivative units joined to form a long, unbranched chain. Chitosan is the N-deacetylated product of chitin. Both chitin and chitosan are main constituents of the exoskeletons of many arthropods. They are also found in structures of invertebrate organisms and the cell walls of most fungi.

Chondroitm Sulfate. Chondroitin sulfate consists of repeating units of glucuronic acid linked to N-acetyl-D-galactosamine. It is a major constituent of various connective tissues and can be found particularly in blood vessels, bone, and cartilage.

Cutin. Cutin is a waxy, water-repellent substance that is the major component of the cuticle, a protective layer covering the plant epidermal cells exposed to the environment above ground.

Degrees of Polymerization. Degrees of polymerization is the number of anhydromonosaccharide units in a polysaccharide.

APPENDIX B

Dextrins. Partial degradation products of starch digestion that are fully digestible in the human small intestine. Sometimes referred to as maltodextrins. Dextrins are not to be confused with resistant maltodextrins.

Fructan. Fructan is a general term for any carbohydrate consisting of linear or branched fructose polymers that constitute the majority of the glycosidic units.

Fructooligosaccharide. See oligofructose.

Galactooligosaccharide. Galactooligosaccharides are nondigestible oligosaccharides (3 to 10 degrees of polymerization) composed of galactose units that escape digestion in the stomach and small intestine and arrive in the colon.

Gums. Gums consist of a diverse group of water soluble polysaccharides usually isolated from seeds and typically viscous in aqueous solution.

Hemicelluloses. Hemicelluloses are a group of polysaccharides found in plant cell walls that surround the cellulose fibers. These polymers can be linear or branched and consist of glucose, arabinose, mannose, xylose, and galacturonic acid.

Hydrocolloid. Synonym for gum (e.g., guar gum, locust bean gum, and gum arabic). Hydrocolloids are widely used in small amounts as food additives to modify textural, water retention, and rehydration properties.

Intact. As used in the definition *of Dietary Fiber*, intact is defined as having no relevant component removed or destroyed (Gove, 1967).

Intrinsic. As used in the definition of *Dietary Fiber*, intrinsic is defined as originating and included wholly within (Gove, 1967).

Inulin. Inulin is a β-(2,1)-linked fructose polymer usually terminated by a glucose unit that was originally isolated from dahlia tubers. It is a naturally occurring component of plants such as chicory and Jerusalem artichoke.

Lectins. Lectins are proteins with sugar-binding sites that can agglutinate cells and/or precipitate molecules that contain carbohydrate.

Lignin. Lignin is a highly-branched polymer comprised of phenylpropanoid units and is found within "woody" plant cell walls, covalently bound to fibrous polysaccharides.

Maillard Reaction Products. Maillard reaction products are produced by one form of nonenzymatic browning in which the carbonyl groups of acyclic sugars interact with free amino groups of amino acids. This occurs when the carbohydrate solution becomes neutral or weakly alkaline, which favors the acyclic carbonyl forms of reducing sugars.

Mixed Linkage β-Glucans. Mixed linkage β-glucans are homopolysaccharides of branched glucose residues. These β-linked D-glucopyranose polymers are constituents of fungi, algae, and higher plants and include mixed linkage β-glucans in cereals.

Modified Cellulose. Modified cellulose is produced by treatment of cellulose fibers, obtained from cotton linters or wood pulp, yielding cellulose derivatives such as methyl ether or hydroxypropyl ether of cellulose.

Mucilage. Mucilage is a thick, viscous plant cell product, and the term is usually applied to plant gums.

Nondigestible. Nondigestible is an adjective that implies a substance is not broken down to simpler chemical compounds in the living body chiefly through the action of secretion-containing enzymes such as the saliva and the gastric, pancreatic, and intestinal juices in the alimentary canal of higher animals (Gove, 1967).

Nonstarch Polysaccharide. Polymeric fraction of fiber that includes all polysaccharides and excludes lignin and all starch. Nonstarch polysaccharide is typically a mixture of cellulose, hemicellulose, pectins, and gums.

Novel Fibre. Health Canada has defined novel fibre as a food that has been manufactured to be a source of dietary fiber and: has not traditionally been used for human consumption to any significant extent; or has been chemically processed (e.g., oxidized) or physically processed (e.g., very finely ground) so as to modify the properties of the fibre; or has been highly concentrated from its plant source. It must be demonstrated that a novel fibre is safe and that it functions physiologically as dietary fiber for it to be considered a source of dietary fiber.

Oligofructose. Oligofructose, also known as fructooligosaccharide, is the hydrolysis product of inulin and consists of 3 to 5 units comprised of fructose with a terminal glucose unit. Oligofructose, which is produced by the action of the fungal enzyme β-fructofuranosidase on inulin, can be found naturally in plants such as onions.

Oligosaccharides. Oligosaccharides are compounds containing 2 to 10 monosaccharides of the same or varying sugar units linked in a linear or branched chain. The division between Oligosaccharides and polysaccharides is somewhat arbitrary, with the upper limit of size for Oligosaccharides varying from 7 to 15 sugar residues. Examples of intrinsic Oligosaccharides are stachyose, raffinose, and verbacose found in legumes and Oligofructose in onions.

Pectins. Pectins, which are found in cell wall and intracellular tissues of many fruits and berries, consist of galacturonic acid units with rhamnose interspersed in a linear chain. Pectins frequently have side chains of neutral sugars, and the galactose units may be esterified with a methyl group, a feature that allows for the viscosity of an aqueous solution of pectin.

Phytate. Phytate (inositol hexaphosphate) is typically found in the outer layers of cereal grains and can decrease the absorption of trace elements in the intestine.

APPENDIX B

Polydex- Polydextrose is a glucose polymer produced under vacuum at a high
trose. temperature in the presence of a food acid catalyst with sorbitol as a
plasticizer. It is commonly used as a bulking agent and sometimes as a
sugar substitute.

Psyllium. Psyllium refers to the husk of psyllium seeds and is a very viscous
mucilage in aqueous solution. The psyllium seed, also known as plantago
or flea seed, is small, dark, reddish-brown, odorless, and nearly tasteless. *P. ovata*, known as blond or Indian plantagoa seed, is the species from which
husk is usually derived. *P. ramosa* is known as Spanish or French psyllium
seed.

Resistant Resistant maltodextrins are largely an indigestible mixture of oligo- and
Maltodex- polysaccharides manufactured by pyrolysis and subsequent enzymatic
trin. treatment of cornstarch.

Resistant Resistant starch comprises starch and starch degradation products not
Starch. digested and absorbed in the small intestine of humans. Resistant starch
consists of starch not physically accessible to digestive enzymes, cooked
starch in granules not accessible to digestion unless the granules are
gelatinized by heating, and retrograded amylose that has been rendered
resistant to enzymatic hydrolysis by processing or by cooking and cooling.

Saponin. Saponin is any plant glycoside that can be hydrolyzed to produce a
carbohydrate and a sapogenin, a steroid or a triterpene component. The
carbohydrate may be glucose, galactose, or a methylpentose.

Sorbitol. Sorbitol is a sugar alcohol formed by reduction of the carbonyl (aldehyde)
group of glucose.

Tannins. Tannins (or tannic acid) occur naturally in many parts of plants including
the roots, wood, bark, leaves, and fruit. They are responsible for the
astringent taste, flavor, and color of many varieties of coffee and tea.

Viscous. A viscous compound is liquid-like but is thick and therefore has a
resistance to flow.

Wax. Waxes are pliable substances that are less greasy, harder, more brittle, and
contain compounds of higher molecular weight than fats. They can
originate from plant, animal, mineral, or synthetic sources.

Appendix C

Development and Evolution of Methods Used to Extract and Measure Dietary Fiber

Two general types of methods have been developed for isolating and analyzing dietary fiber: enzymatic-gravimetric and enzymatic-chemical. The food components isolated vary depending on the method used. Both the enzymatic-gravimetric and enzymatic-chemical methods have undergone a number of modifications and improvements, most occurring over the last 20 years. The enzymatic-gravimetric approach attempts to reflect the material that enters the large intestine by removing starch, protein, and fat and obtaining a residue that is then dried and weighed. A correction is made for any remaining protein and ash, and the result is expressed as a proportion of the starting material. The enzymatic-chemical approach chemically characterizes the carbohydrate content of fiber after the removal of available carbohydrate (monosaccharides, disaccharides, and starch) and fat. A number of different procedures have been developed to enable carbohydrates to be measured as their constituent monosaccharides or as groups of monosaccharide types. The current available methods and their various formats and major modifications are outlined in Table 2 and Table 4.

ENZYMATIC-GRAVIMETRIC METHODS

The gravimetric approach began with the measurement of crude fiber, developed at the Weende Research Station in Germany in the latter half of the nineteenth century (Henneberg and Stohmann, 1860). The method comprised of treatment of plant material with acid and alkali, resulting in a residue. The method became well established during the early part of the twentieth century, and a modification of the original method was later adopted by the Association of Official Analytical Chemists International (AOAC) as a method for measuring fiber in animal feeds (AOAC, 1995). The crude fiber method was used for the determination of the fiber content for the U.S. Food Composition tables in the 1970s (Watt, 1976). It continues to be used in some regions of the world as well as the animal feed industry. However, its usefulness is severely limited by the loss of all soluble polysaccharides, some insoluble polysaccharides, and some lignin, and the inclusion of some nitrogenous material in the remaining residue.

In the 1960s, Van Soest and colleagues introduced the use of detergents to solubilize protein. The Acid Detergent Fiber (ADF) method, which was adopted for animal feeds, utilizes strong acid to hydrolyze all polysaccharides except cellulose and lignin, which are therefore the only components in ADF (Van Soest, 1963). Other cell wall polysaccharides are not included in this method, limiting its usefulness for human nutrition in the same way as crude fiber.

Recognizing the need to describe and include other cell wall constituents, Van Soest and Wine (1967) developed the Neutral Detergent Fiber (NDF) method, which measures all insoluble cell wall material. This proved to be a better predictor of the nutritional value of dietary fiber in animal feeds than crude fiber. In the 1970s, the use of the NDF method spread to human nutrition, but its utility remained limited because it did not include soluble fiber components nor did it remove all starch.

With growing interest in dietary fiber in human nutrition in the 1970s and the development of a physiological role for this dietary component, there was a need for an analytical method that measured insoluble cell wall and soluble fiber components. German researchers introduced the use of enzymes during the nineteenth century to remove available carbohydrate, and this approach was used by Williams and Olmsted (1935) in the United States in an effort to measure the indigestible material in a more physiological way in their human studies. Building on this work, a number of investigators, such as Asp and Johansson (1981), Furda (1977), Hellendoorn and colleagues (1975), and Schweizer and Würsch (1979), developed analytical approaches that reflected the "nondigested" fraction of the diet, including soluble material as well as insoluble components. Prosky and coworkers (1985) published a method that was based on the work of these various investigators, and it was subsequently adopted by AOAC as AOAC method 985.29. The method provides a measure of total dietary fiber by enzymatic removal of available starch and solubilization and extraction of a portion of the protein; the remaining residue is dried, weighed, and corrected for crude protein and ash contents. An initial step is added to remove fat if it is present at concentrations of 10 percent or more. The method is relatively rapid and easy to perform and has been automated to enable a large number of samples to be assessed. It has been adopted as an official method for dietary fiber analysis by many countries.

The method was extended to the determination of soluble and insoluble dietary fiber as the need to measure these components was recognized (Prosky et al., 1988, 1992, 1994). Other related methods were subsequently validated by AOAC collaborative studies and approved as official by AOAC. Lee and co-workers (1992) substituted MES-TRIS buffer in place of the original phosphate buffer, and in doing so, generated the new AOAC method 991.43. Li and Cardozo (1994) introduced a simpler method (AOAC method 993.21) for foods that contain little or no starch, such as fruits and some vegetables. Mongeau and Brassard (1993) took a somewhat different approach, using a modified NDF method to measure insoluble fiber and a new approach to analyze for the soluble fiber fraction (AOAC method 992.16).

As shown in Table 4, there are two ways of deriving soluble fiber: (1) by direct analysis (Mongeau and Brassard, 1993), and (2) by subtraction of insoluble fiber from total fiber (Englyst and Hudson, 1987; Quigley and Englyst, 1992).

ENZYMATIC-CHEMICAL METHODS

It was recognized early on that significant proportions of the carbohydrate, which are resistant to human digestive enzymes, are soluble in nature and lost when fiber is recovered by filtration. McCance and Lawrence (1929) developed a method for "unavailable carbohydrates" which involved reflux with strong acid, followed by colorimetric determination of reducing sugars and pentoses.

During the 1950s, Southgate continued to develop this chemical approach to fiber measurement, extending McCance and Lawrence's work by introducing a series of extraction steps followed by hydrolysis of polysaccharides and subsequent colorimetric analysis of component monosaccharides. He published his procedure for unavailable carbohydrates in 1969 (Southgate, 1969). Southgate recognized that a crucial step was the complete removal of starch since incomplete removal would result in overestimation of glucose-based dietary fiber. The Southgate method was modified for human nutrition during the 1970s and became incorporated in the United Kingdom nutrient tables in the Fourth Edition of McCance and Widdowson's *The Composition of Foods* (Paul and Southgate, 1978).

Although the method provided considerable information on monosaccharide groups (hexoses, pentoses, and uronic acids), Southgate recognized that a colorimetric assay did not distinguish individual monosaccharides, and recommended that gas chromatography (GC) or high-performance liquid chromatography (HPLC) be employed (Southgate, 1981). In addition, there remained difficulties with the removal of starch, which gave inflated values for many individual food items with high starch content such as starchy vegetables, legumes, and grains. Englyst and coworkers (1982) published a procedure extending Southgate's work for the measurement of nonstarch polysaccharides using GC. The method in volved more complete removal of available starch and allowed for determination of the different monosaccharides present as constituents of dietary fiber in food products. It also allowed for separation of cellulose from noncellulosic polysaccharides, and soluble from insoluble polysaccharides. Hence, the method provided considerable detail on the polysaccharide components of human foods.

Several modifications have been made to the 1982 Englyst method. One of these was the removal of resistant starch, which was identified in the early 1980s (Englyst and Cummings, 1984). Resistant starch consists of (1) starch that is not physically accessible to digestive enzymatic hydrolysis; (2) retrograded starch that has been rendered resistant to hydrolysis by processing or by cooking and cooling; and (3) uncooked starch in granules that is not accessible to enzymatic hydrolysis unless it is gelatinized by heating (Englyst et al., 1992a). Englyst and Cummings (1984) removed resistant starch from the nonstarch polysaccharide component in a method using dimethyl sulfoxide. Since resistant starch is created by cooking and processing, the method ensured that foods could be assessed using nonstarch polysaccharide values of ingredients by the use of recipes, and that each food product did not have to be individually measured to obtain an accurate value.

In response to criticism that the method was too time consuming, Englyst and Hudson (1987) developed an alternative colorimetric method for the measurement of the component monosaccharides. Englyst made the procedure faster in another modification, with a more rapid procedure for the removal of starch (Englyst et al., 1992b). HPLC methods were developed for the measurement of uronic acids (Englyst et al., 1994; Quigley and Englyst, 1994).

Prior to Englyst's work, Theander and Åman (1979) developed a chemical method that used GC to measure soluble and insoluble fiber components. This method was later modified to improve starch hydrolysis (Theander and Westerlund, 1986) and to measure the fiber-derived monosaccharides by HPLC (Shinnick et al., 1988). The procedure does not remove resistant starch and measures lignin separately as Klason lignin, material insoluble in 72 percent sulfuric acid (Goering and Van Soest, 1970). Originally, the method did not rely on ethanol precipitation of solubilized fiber components, but rather recovered them from the soluble fraction by dialysis with a molecular weight cutoff of 12,000 to 14,000 daltons. Subsequently, the procedure was simplified and made more rapid by precipitating solubilized fiber components with 80 percent ethanol (Theander et al., 1994).

COMPONENTS INCLUDED IN EACH METHOD OF ANALYSIS

A list of potential components of fiber included or not included in each analysis is provided in Table 2.

Nonstarch Polysaccharides

All the current methods include all nonstarch polysaccharides that precipitate in 78 to 80 percent ethanol. Polysaccharides that do not precipitate in ethanol are not included in any of the existing methods. Polysaccharides that are excluded by ethanol precipitation include inulin, other fructans, modified cellulose, and some arabinogalactans.

Lignin

All methods except those of Englyst (Englyst and Cummings, 1984; Englyst and Hudson, 1987; Quigley and Englyst, 1992) for nonstarch polysaccharides include lignin. In the enzymatic-gravimetric methods, this is included as part of the residue after filtration. In the enzymatic-chemical methods of Theander and coworkers (1994) and Southgate (1969), it is analyzed as a separate component, using the Klason lignin method (Goering and Van Soest, 1970). This method measures native lignin, but can also include tannins, cutins, and Maillard reaction products (Theander et al., 1995).

Resistant Starch

Resistant starch is not included in the Englyst methods for nonstarch polysaccharides (Englyst and Cummings, 1984; Englyst and Hudson, 1987; Quigley and Englyst, 1992), since it is removed using dimethyl sulfoxide. In all the other methods, a proportion of resistant starch is included in the analysis for dietary fiber, largely as retrograded amylose. However, this proportion of resistant starch is not constant for different foods made from the same ingredients, as retrograded amylose is created by cooking and cooling food and through food processing. Since resistant starch has many physiological properties similar to those of dietary fiber, there is a need for a uniform method for its analysis.

There are currently a number of methods available for measurement of resistant starch, although none have been submitted for evaluation by the approved methods process of the AOAC. Several of these were developed during the European Resistant Starch (EURESTA) program which involved 40 research groups in 11 countries, all involved in resistant starch research from 1990 to 1995 (Asp et al., 1996). Björck and colleagues (1986) reported the starch remaining in the dietary fiber residue from the Asp enzymatic-gravimetric procedure, using potassium hydroxide (Asp et al., 1983). Englyst and colleagues (1992a) calculated resistant starch as the difference between available starch and total starch. Muir and O'Dea (1992) developed a method based on more physiological influences, as did Åkerberg and colleagues (1998).

TABLE 4 Methods of Fiber Analysis

Reference (Method)	Procedure Type	Measures
Asp et al., 1983	Enzymatic-gravimetric	Soluble dietary fiber Insoluble dietary fiber Total dietary fiber
Craig et al., 2000 (AOAC 2000.11)	Enzymatic-ion exchange chromatographic	Polydextrose
Englyst and Cummings, 1984	Enzymatic-gas chromatographic	Total nonstarch polysaccharides Individual constituent sugars
Englyst and Hudson, 1987	Enzymatic-colorimetric	Soluble nonstarch polysaccharides, by difference Insoluble nonstarch polysaccharides Total nonstarch polysaccharides
Gordon and Ohkuma, in press (AOAC 2001.03)	Enzymatic-gravimetric liquid chromatographic	Total dietary fiber including low molecular weight resistant maltodextrins
Hoebregs, 1997 (AOAC 997.08)	Enzymatic-ion exchange chromatographic	Fructans
Lee et al., 1992 (AOAC 991.43)	Enzymatic-gravimetric using MES-TRIS buffer	Soluble dietary fiber Insoluble dietary fiber Total dietary fiber
Li and Cardozo, 1994 (AOAC 993.21)	Enzymatic-gravimetric (For foods and food products with ≤ 2% starch)	Total dietary fiber
McCleary et al., 2000 (AOAC 999.03)	Enzymatic-spectrophotometric	Fructans
Mongeau and Brassard, 1993 (AOAC 992.16)	Enzymatic-gravimetric	Soluble dietary fiber Insoluble dietary fiber Total dietary fiber
Prosky et al., 1985	Enzymatic-gravimetric	Total dietary fiber
Prosky et al., 1992 (AOAC 991.42)	Enzymatic-gravimetric	Insoluble dietary fiber

APPENDIX C

Total Dietary Fiber Determination	Concerns
Calculated as the weight of fiber residue less the weight of protein and ash or calculated as the sum of soluble and insoluble fiber	
Not applicable	
Calculated as the sum of the monosaccharides	Does not estimate lignin
Sum of hexoses, pentoses, and uronic acids	Does not estimate lignin
Calculated as the sum of insoluble fiber, high molecular weight and low molecular weight soluble fibers	
Not applicable	
Measured by independent analysis or calculated as the sum of soluble fiber and insoluble fiber	
Calculated as the weight of fiber residue less the weight of protein and ash	
Not applicable	
Calculated as the sum of the soluble and insoluble fiber	
Calculated as the weight of fiber residue less the weight of protein and ash	
Not applicable	

APPENDIX C

Reference (Method)	Procedure Type	Measures
Prosky et al., 1994 (AOAC 993.19)	Enzymatic-gravimetric	Soluble dietary fiber
Quigley and Englyst, 1992	Enzymatic-high performance liquid chromatographic	Soluble nonstarch polysaccharides, by difference Insoluble nonstarch polysaccharides Total nonstarch polysaccharides Individual constituent sugars
Schweizer and Würsch, 1979	Enzymatic-gravimetric	Soluble dietary fiber Insoluble dietary fiber Total dietary fiber
Southgate, 1969	Enzymatic-colorimetric	Soluble dietary fiber Insoluble dietary fiber Total dietary fiber
Theander and Åman, 1979	Enzymatic-gas chromatographic	Insoluble neutral polysaccharides Soluble neutral polysaccharides Insoluble uronic acids Soluble uronic acids Klason lignin Total dietary fiber
Theander and Westerlund, 1986	Enzymatic-gas chromatographic	Insoluble neutral polysaccharides Soluble neutral polysaccharides Insoluble uronic acids Soluble uronic acids Klason lignin Total dietary fiber
Uppsala Method of Theander et al., 1995 (AOAC 994.13)	Enzymatic-gas chromatographic	Neutral polysaccharides Uronic acids Klason lignin Total dietary fiber

Total Dietary Fiber Determination	Concerns
Not applicable	
Calculated as the sum of the monosaccharides	Does not estimate lignin
Calculated as the sum of soluble and insoluble fiber	
Sum of hexoses, pentoses, uronic acids, and lignin	Incomplete removal of starch; not specific with respect to individual sugars (Theander and Westerlund, 1986)
Calculated as the sum of neutral polysaccharides, uronic acids, and Klason lignin	
Calculated as the sum of neutral polysaccharides, uronic acids, and Klason lignin	
Calculated as the sum of neutral polysaccharide residues, uronic acid residues, and Klason lignin	

Champ (1992) has published a method based on extensive use of amylase, resulting in a direct method for resistant starch, rather than by difference of total starch and residual starch. More recently, McCleary (2001b) modified and simplified the method (AOAC method 996.11) of Goñi and colleagues (1996), which closely reflects conditions in the small intestine. Comparisons between methods tend to produce similar results, although not for all types of foods (Champ et al., 2001; McCleary, 2001a). Digestion and absorption in the human gastrointestinal tract is a dynamic process in which many enzymes, including proteases and amylases, work in concert to disrupt the three dimensional and then the intermolecular relationships in foods. Macromolecules are hydrolyzed as they become exposed, and hydrolytic products are rapidly absorbed. The successful analytical method for resistant starch will be one that mimics this process in the human gastrointestinal tract, so that the analytically determined value reflects starch not assimilated in the human.

Oligosaccharides

Compounds of chain length less than 10 monosaccharide units are generally soluble in 78 to 80 percent ethanol, do not precipitate, and are not included in any of the analytical methods for dietary fiber. However, many of these behave physiologically in a similar way to polysaccharides, and hence there has been a need to analyze for them. Quigley and Englyst (1992) published an HPLC method for Oligosaccharides from a number of sources, and methods have also been or are currently being developed for specific Oligosaccharides, such as fructooligosaccharides (Hoebregs, 1997; McCleary and Blakeney, 1999; McCleary et al., 2000), and galactooligosaccharides (de Slegte, in press). The method for galactooligosaccharides has received AOAC approval (AOAC method 2001.02).

Fructans, Inulin, and Oligofructose

Inulin, a polymer of fructose found in a small number of vegetables, fruit, and grains, is soluble in 78 to 80 percent ethanol and is therefore not detected by any of the currently AOAC approved dietary fiber methods. The hydrolysis product of inulin is oligofructose, also called fructooligosaccharide, and is similarly soluble in ethanol and not included as fiber by any method for fiber analysis. Because of widespread interest in these compounds, a number of methods have been developed for their measurement in foods (Hoebregs, 1997; McCleary and Blakeney, 1999; McCleary et al., 2000). These entail hydrolysis to fructose and glucose, which are then measured by a variety of methods.

Polydextrose

Polydextrose is a synthesized polysaccharide created by thermal polymerization of glucose. It is not precipitated with 78 to 80 percent ethanol and is therefore not included in the analysis of dietary fiber by any of the existing methods. There are specific methods for the analysis of polydextrose, which have been developed and improved since the development of the polysaccharide. Of these, the most comprehensive is that using HPLC, which has recently gained AOAC approval (AOAC method 2000.11) (Craig et al., 2000).

Modified Cellulose

There are a number of modified cellulose compounds, such as methyl cellulose, carboxymethyl cellulose, and derivatives of these, which are soluble and do not precipitate in 78 to 80 percent ethanol. Several of these compounds are used as laxative agents and in a variety of food products such as salad dressings, icings and toppings, desserts, and baked goods (Sandford and Baird, 1983). They have many of the same physiological properties as dietary fiber.

Resistant Maltodextrins

Resistant maltodextrins are produced through various acid/pressure processes, are not susceptible to enzymatic hydrolysis, and have similar properties to fiber, but they do not precipitate in 78 to 80 percent ethanol and are therefore not included in any current analytical method for dietary fiber. Currently, there is an enzymatic-gravimetric-liquid chromatographic method for the analysis of resistant maltodextrins, and the method of Gordon and Ohkuma (in press) has gained the approval of the AOAC for its analysis (AOAC method 2001.03).

Chitin and Chitosan

Chitin and chitosan are polysaccharide-containing materials with chemical structures similar to cellulose and are derived mainly from the outer shell of crab and other sea creatures. Because of the high polysaccharide content, these materials may have physiological properties similar to dietary fiber. Some of these compounds are insoluble in 78 to 80 percent ethanol and therefore analyze as dietary fiber by all current dietary fiber methods. However, the proportion of the total that can be analyzed as dietary fiber depends on the manner and extent of processing of the source material prior to analysis.

Chondroitin

Chondroitin and chondroitin sulfate are polysaccharide-containing compounds found in connective tissues of animals, particularly blood vessels, bone, and cartilage. Some of these compounds precipitate in 78 to 80 percent ethanol and therefore analyze as dietary fiber by current methods.

Noncarbohydrate Components

Because of the nonspecific nature of the gravimetric methods, these methods include components that are not carbohydrate. Hence, the methods of Lee (Lee et al., 1992), Mongeau and Brassard (1993), Prosky (Prosky et al., 1985, 1988, 1992, 1994), and earlier versions of any of these include lignin, cutin, tannins, and Maillard reaction products as well as other less well-characterized compounds. The contribution of these components in most unrefined foods is very small, but processing can increase their presence through complexing in various ways. Maillard reaction products, for example, are generated through heating, and therefore application of heat through processing or cooking will increase their contribution to dietary fiber content. However, in most instances the increase in dietary fiber content caused by heat-generated Maillard reaction products is insignificant. The enzymatic-chemical methods of Englyst (Englyst and Cummings, 1984; Englyst and Hudson, 1987; Quigley and Englyst, 1992), Southgate (1969), and Theander (Theander and Åman, 1979; Theander and Westerlund, 1986; Theander et al., 1995) do not include these noncarbohydrate components in the analysis of polysaccharides because these procedures analyze carbohydrate directly. However, Klason lignin included in the dietary fiber values obtained by the Theander methods (Theander and Åman, 1979; Theander and Westerlund, 1986; Theander et al., 1995) include some tannins and Maillard reaction products.

SUMMARY

In some countries, isolated/purified fibers are specified as dietary fiber if they analyze as dietary fiber by the accepted fiber methods. Examples of substances that have been extracted from plant materials include cellulose, hemicellulose, gums, and pectins. These have traditionally been considered dietary fiber and are captured in the existing dietary fiber methods. Other unabsorbable carbohydrates have been chemically synthesized or made resistant through physical or chemical modifications and include resistant starch, resistant malto-dextrin, polydextrose, and hydroxymethylcellulose. Some of these synthesized compounds may also appear naturally in foods, such as resistant starch. Other unavailable carbohydrates that may have physiological effects, such as inulin, are not measured by most accepted dietary fiber methods and have not been included as dietary fiber. The technology is available to synthesize an infinite number of these food components. Unavailable carbohydrates with fiber-like properties may be manufactured de novo, modified, or isolated from existing fiber sources for incorporation into foods or supplements. The challenge of defining dietary fiber is that potential sources that may either meet chemical definitions or physiological endpoint requirements are expanding at a fast rate and challenge the existing methods to determine fiber.

APPENDIX C

Appendix D
Determination Of Energy Values For Fibers

A side issue related to how dietary fiber is defined is how its contribution to food energy is determined. Exact values for digestible, metabolizable, and net energy of fibers are difficult to determine. Differences in food composition, patterns of food consumption, the administered dose of fiber, the metabolic status of the individual (i.e., obese, lean, malnourished, etc.), and digestive capabilities of individuals influence the digestible energy consumed and the metabolizable energy available from various dietary fibers. Similarly, individual variation in physical and metabolic activities affects net energy. In addition, interspecies differences from basic research studies, the variety of analytical methods used, the numerous experimental variables tested, and the variation in standard operating procedures used by investigators make data interpretation difficult and hamper the determination of exact values for metabolizable energy and net energy from dietary fiber. Finally, the amount of carbon from dietary fiber that ends up as microbial matter and the nutrient trapping effect (i.e., more protein and fat are excreted in feces as a result of dietary fiber ingestion) affect the results obtained.

Despite these complexities, approximate values or ranges of values sufficiently accurate for regulatory purposes have been derived from available data. These values should be viewed with caution because many experimental animal studies and human clinical trials from which energy values are taken have differences in protocol design and conduct that make statistical analysis and comparisons difficult.

Several methods exist to determine the energy concentration of dietary fibers. These were reviewed by Fahey and Grieshop (2000) and include gross energy determination, energy balance method, factorial calculation of the metabolizable energy value, calculation of the net energy of maintenance, indirect calorimetry, breath hydrogen determination, and radiolabel technique.

Because the process of fermentation is anaerobic, less energy is recovered from dietary fiber than the 4 kcal/g obtained from aerobic glycolysis. Fermentation balance equations and molar ratios of short chain fatty acids in human stool can be used to estimate that anaerobic metabolism yields 2 to 3 kcal/g of hexose fermented (Hungate, 1966; Miller and Wolin, 1979), a calculation that assumed that short chain fatty acids were actively absorbed from the large intestine and that those generated by one strain of bacteria were not utilized by another microbial species.

Available data suggest that neither of these assumptions apply. It appears that the short-chain fatty acid, propionate, is utilized by some bacteria and is, therefore, unavailable for absorption. Also, data suggest that in monogastric species, short-chain fatty acids are passively absorbed from the large intestine, meaning that only when the concentration is greater in the colonic lumen than in the adjacent tissue does absorption occur (Fleming and Yeo, 1990).

Absorption of short-chain fatty acids is closely linked to the movement of water and electrolytes from the lumen, and participation in the normal secretory and absorption activities in the colon is one of the important physiological functions of short-chain fatty acids (Argenzio et al., 1975). Short-chain fatty acids are the main anions in human feces (Høverstad et al., 1984). Although this has not been well documented, humans, in contrast to most animals that consume highly defined diets, consume excess electrolytes and protein, the latter requiring ample buffering capacity. The role of short-chain fatty acids in electrolyte and acid-base balance undoubtedly dominates over their absorption and subsequent use as an energy source. Therefore, it is not possible for anaerobic fermentation to generate 4 kcal/g, and it is unlikely that the theoretical yield of 3 kcal/g is absorbed from the large intestine. Indeed, data indicate that the average energy yield from dietary fiber fermentation in monogastric species is in the range of 1.5 to 2.5 kcal/g (Livesey, 1990; Smith et al., 1998).